PROMISE AND PERFORMANCE
IN MANAGED CARE

T0146278

PROMISE AND PERFORMANCE IN MANAGED CARE

The Prepaid Group Practice Model

**Donald K. Freeborn
and Clyde R. Pope**

Center for Health Research
Kaiser Permanente, Northwest Region

The Johns Hopkins University Press
Baltimore and London

© 1994 The Johns Hopkins University Press
All rights reserved. Published 1994
Printed in the United States of America on acid-free paper
03 02 01 00 99 98 97 96 95 94   5 4 3 2 1

The Johns Hopkins University Press
2715 North Charles Street
Baltimore, Maryland 21218-4319
The Johns Hopkins Press Ltd., London

Library of Congress Cataloging-in-Publication Data
will be found at the end of this book.

ISBN 0-8018-4819-9

A catalog record for this book is available from the British Library.

ISBN 0-8018-6360-0 (pbk)
paperback edition, 1999

Contents

Foreword   vii

Acknowledgments   xi

Introduction   1

1   The Rise of Managed Care   12

2   Choosing a Managed Care Plan   28

3   Access and Continuity in Managed Care   51

4   Patient Satisfaction with Managed Care   70

5   Physician Satisfaction with Managed Care   93

6   The Future of Managed Care   120

Appendix: Data Sources, Survey Design and Analysis, and
Multivariate Tables   139

References   147

Index   167

Foreword

The appearance of this monograph, *Promise and Performance in Managed Care,* would be valuable at any time, but it has particular significance coming as it does after the release of the health care reform plan by the Clinton administration and the debate over components of the proposal. Prepared largely before specific elements of health care reform were laid out, the book identifies and discusses issues that have been the object of sharp debate, both those on which there is a great deal of agreement and those on which sharp disagreements made it unlikely that a bill would be passed quickly.

From the beginning, several provisions of the Clinton plan have been widely accepted: coverage of the unemployed and the poorly insured by a comprehensive package of health care benefits; community rating, meaning the end of differential pricing and restrictions that have existed in health insurance for the chronically ill and others with disability; reduced paperwork; and emphasis on managed care. The criticisms most often heard relate to the cost of the program and proposed cost-control measures, poorly understood details of benefits and gaps, the organization and operation of the system, the scope of choice of the source of care, and the advantages of a single-payer program.

Attracting too little attention are the components calling for a uniform system of reporting services or bills, and the development of methods for evaluating the quality and outcome of care that far exceed the methods and systems we have today. And yet, these activities have the prospect of creating important sources of information for inquiries on the delivery of care, and for health care research affecting all ages and ethnic groups. None of this will happen quickly, but for those of us who can look back twenty-five years or more and recall the fits and starts of similar ventures on a smaller geographic scale and a narrower age basis, the critical issue is to initiate the process well. This requires forethought regarding the questions the data systems need to answer by themselves or in connection with the information systems of the National Center for Health Statistics. It also requires research on cost effectiveness, the appropriateness of clinical practice, and patient outcomes, like that currently funded by the Agency for Health Care Policy and Research. Finally, the data systems and research need to respond to questions raised by other agencies at the national and state levels.

An object lesson can be found in the Medicare system, from which we have learned a great deal but which has a built-in age restriction (except for the relatively small disability group covered). But we should not overlook the relevance to current and future problems of the steps taken by a few health insurance plans, an outstanding example of which is the Kaiser Permanente (KP) Center for Health Research. Indeed, we should be thankful that we now have a volume made possible by a long-term investment in information systems that seek to answer questions about the KP plan's functioning that are useful to both insiders and outsiders.

Mitch Greenlick and Ernie Saward, the first research director and first medical director, respectively, of Kaiser Permanente, Northwest Region, saw the need for a continuous, systematic assessment of how a comprehensive prepaid group practice functions, with insights into its strengths and problems. They introduced a sampling scheme for ambulatory care, total coverage of hospitalizations, and periodic surveys of the membership (utilizers and nonutilizers) and the community at large, out of which flowed a large stream of publications.

In this monograph, Don Freeborn and Clyde Pope examine the potential for HMOs of the group practice variety to deliver managed care, and some of the consequences. Statements are supported by the data derived from special research data systems, from the KP plan's information system, and from observations by other researchers, including those prominently associated with the formulation of health policy. The context is the long-term operation of a plan based on principles that are advanced by the authors as incorporating desirable features of managed care.

As popular as the term *managed care* is, professionals in the field vary in their definitions of it. When examined from the population's standpoint, it should signify the commitment of a plan to primary care, the continuity and coordination of health care, access to care, and the effort to improve the outcome of care and to plan and deliver preventive services. However, from a management standpoint, economically driven characteristics dictate what managed care is. As Freeborn and Pope point out, these include contractual arrangements with providers to furnish comprehensive services (often on a capitation basis), the acceptance of utilization- and quality-control measures by the providers, and financial incentives to patients and providers for appropriate use of the system. Obviously the two ideas overlap, but, depending on which is emphasized and practiced, the general public and providers may decide differently what type of health plan should be selected and stayed with over the long run.

Group practice HMOs are viewed as a model of how a plan can best realize desirable features of managed care—including the provision of preventive, diagnostic, and therapeutic services in an integrated program—and achieve cost control. Many of the ideas will be familiar. After all, we have heard about this type of HMO for years. The difference is the marshalling of information on a well-established, successful program in a period when, as a matter of national policy, HMOs are apparently favored. A single program is assessed, but we can view the experience as telling us what can be achieved rather than as a description of how HMOs in general function today.

This monograph provides us with a perspective that is well worth attending to. Freeborn and Pope reexamine many questions that have been raised about the HMO variety of managed care and then interpret the policy implications of what they have found. The scope is large, including an exploration of why people select alternative plans and why they stay with or move away from them; an examination of personal and system factors that influence the utilization of services; a comparison of individuals' satisfaction with various aspects of the HMO program and similar judgments regarding the fee-for-service source of care; and a study of physicians attitudes and of what physicians like and dislike about the HMO.

Some readers, taking the data and the arguments as one-sided, will have complaints (e.g., that the lower levels of satisfaction among patients of HMOs are inadequately considered; that the clinical practice and financial controls exercised by HMOs are more serious than described and will deter many physicians from entering such programs; and that the favorable economic status achieved by many HMOs is due to the enrollment of low utilizers). Freeborn and Pope weigh the problems of patients and physicians and discount the charge that HMOs give preference in enrollment to healthier groups. For many readers, the advantages and disadvantages will represent a balanced view of what is achievable in managed care directed by a well-functioning HMO.

Sam Shapiro
Professor Emeritus and Acting Chair
Department of Health Policy and Management
The Johns Hopkins School of Hygiene and Public Health

Acknowledgments

We required the assistance of many people to produce this book, but we would never have written it had it not been for Merwyn R. (Mitch) Greenlick, who provided the commitment, energy, and leadership that transformed the vision of a prepaid group practice–based research program into the Center for Health Research (CHR), a nationally recognized institution conducting research in the public interest. For this reason, and because of the tremendous intellectual contribution he has made to our individual research endeavors over the years of our association with him, not to mention our great affection for him, we dedicate this book to Mitch.

We also gratefully acknowledge the access we have had to Kaiser Permanente, Northwest Region (KPNW), which has been the research laboratory for investigators at the Center for Health Research since the CHR was established nearly thirty years ago. We appreciate the Northwest Region's support of public domain research and its respect for the CHR's professional and scientific autonomy. Because of this autonomy, the region does not review and approve the publications of CHR investigators. We therefore take sole responsibility for the contents of this book, including our findings and conclusions. We thank those Kaiser Permanente administrators, managers, staff members, and employees who over the years have provided insight and assistance to our research work.

We also recognize with thanks those KPNW members and Northwest Permanente physicians who made this book possible by their participation in our surveys. We are very grateful for their investment of time and energy. Most of the financial support for the membership and physician surveys was provided through grants from the Kaiser Foundation Health Plan of the Northwest and the Community Services Program of Kaiser

Foundation Hospitals, and we gratefully acknowledge this support.

Among others who contributed in some way to the book are those many CHR employees who simply went about doing their jobs well. Over the years, these have included too many people to name. Nevertheless, they know who they are, and we recognize and appreciate their contributions.

Then there are those people we can acknowledge by name, which we do with pleasure. A long-time associate who has participated in various ways in the creation and maintenance of the research capital for our research is Sylvia Marks. In addition to her many other contributions, Ms. Marks worked closely with Clyde Pope in the creation of the KPNW membership surveys, first as a research associate and, since the mid-1970s, as project director for the annual membership surveys and the medical office visit surveys, which began in 1991. The membership surveys have provided much of the data for the chapters on health plan choice and patient satisfaction. We greatly appreciate Ms. Marks's valuable assistance over many years.

Will Mowe, now a health care administrator in Portland, came to the CHR several years ago as a graduate intern from Harvard. He worked with Clyde Pope, and his major project was to review the literature on health plan choice, which was very useful for our chapter on choice of managed care. We acknowledge, with great appreciation, his contribution.

Mark Hornbrook, a health economist and senior investigator at the CHR, worked with Dr. Pope to plan and carry out a community survey on health insurance and health plan choice, which provided much of the empirical data for our chapter on choice. His extensive knowledge of risk assessment, risk adjustment, and the determinants of health plan choice is widely recognized and helped stimulate our thinking for this book. We are grateful for his intellectual contributions and for his support as an esteemed colleague.

Benjamin J. Darsky, a professor (now retired) of medical care organization from the University of Michigan, played a key role in our studies of physicians and, along with Donald Freeborn, designed the CHR's first physician survey in 1977. His rich research experience and extensive knowledge about physicians in organized settings were invaluable, and we simply could not have carried out the research without his assistance. He also served as a consultant to the CHR in its early years and helped design a number of our research data systems. We are indebted to him for his intellectual contributions to our work and for his strong support of the CHR over many years.

We are also pleased to acknowledge the contributions of Harvey

Klevit, a Northwest Permanente (NWP) pediatrician for more than twenty years, a former chief of pediatrics in NWP, and the NWP assistant regional medical director at the time of the 1991 physician survey. Dr. Klevit is now the medical director for the Oregon State Board of Medical Examiners. He made many practical as well as intellectual contributions to the 1991 physician survey, and his efforts made it possible to achieve a high response rate. We greatly benefited from his wisdom and insights about physicians and medical practice in HMOs and other organized settings.

We also acknowledge the contributions of Ralph Schmoldt, a research associate at the CHR during the time this book was being written. Dr. Schmoldt served as project director for the 1991 physician survey and assisted in various ways in the production of the book. In addition to helping design the physician questionnaire, he made substantial contributions to the chapter on physician satisfaction. He also reviewed several of the other chapters.

Valuable research assistance was provided by Vicky Burnham, a long-time CHR employee. Ms. Burnham has played a significant role in all of our physician surveys, as well as in several of our surveys of patient satisfaction. She performed much of the data analysis and supervised the production process for the figures and tables. We greatly appreciate her outstanding and meticulous work, and her dedication to this project. We also recognize the able assistance of Pierre LaChance, a research associate at the CHR, who assisted in organizing and analyzing the utilization data for the chapter on access and continuity of care.

Diann Triebwasser provided excellent secretarial support with patience and good humor through seemingly interminable drafts. Nancy Hunt and Linda Capps assisted by running down many hard-to-find articles, books, and other works, and by performing the painstaking task of checking references for completeness and accuracy.

Gary Miranda, a technical editor at the CHR, reviewed our early drafts and made valiant efforts to help us clarify our ideas, straighten out our prose, and in general improve the organization and readability of the book. His contributions were beyond those usually expected of a technical editor. For this, we are grateful.

Finally, we would like to take this opportunity to thank our wives, Johnni and Lois, for their unwavering support throughout our careers, and for their love and patience during the times we felt most overcome by the demands of this one of our too many projects. We know they will be gentle critics!

Introduction

Toto, I don't think we're in Kansas anymore.
—Dorothy, in *The Wizard of Oz*

Most Americans feel that the U.S. health care system needs fundamental reform (Blendon 1989). Costs continue their upward spiral and access problems become more severe, as the number of people without health insurance increases dramatically (Foley 1992). Despite huge increases in health care spending during the 1980s, both access to health services and the comprehensiveness of benefits declined. The quality of care has deteriorated for many segments of the population, particularly the poor and the near poor (Davis 1991). In spite of the increase in expenditures for health care (from 7% of the gross domestic product in 1970 to 14% in 1993), many question whether the increased spending on health services is significantly improving the health status of the U.S. population (Banta 1990a).

These concerns about the health care system are reflected in current debates, proposed legislation, and health policy recommendations. The central issues are the cost and quality of services and whether services are distributed according to need. The United States spends more on health care per person than any other nation in the world, yet more than 37 million U.S. citizens have no health insurance (USGAO 1991; Rice 1992). Although the United States is one of the wealthiest nations in the world and has developed a medical technology to provide high-quality care, it has not been able to develop an efficient system of delivering health care, and many Americans do not get even minimally adequate health care (Cockerham 1992). High rates of inflation in medical costs, and the excessive use of expensive procedures (which has provided only limited improvement in health outcomes), continue to drive up costs (Banta 1990a). Lack of equity plays a major role in how poor our health care outcomes seem when compared with those of other nations (Davis 1991).

These seemingly intractable problems have led to intensified interest in a variety of strategies to improve the performance of the U.S. health care system. Many health care analysts, third-party payers, and policy makers believe that managed care is the most promising strategy for dealing with the problems of the health care system (Rosko and Broyles 1988; Davis et al. 1990; Iglehart 1992a). But what is managed care? One book on the topic defines managed health care as "any system that manages the delivery of health care in such a way that cost is controlled" (Kongstvedt 1989, xiii). The American Medical Association defines managed care as "the control of access to and limitation on physician and patient utilization of services by public or private payers or their agents through the use of prior and concurrent review for approval of or referral to service or site of service, and financial incentives or penalties" (Iglehart 1992b, 965).

Peter Fox, a health care consultant, provides another definition:

> Broadly defined, [managed care] encompasses any measure that, from the perspective of the purchaser of health care, favorably affects the price of services, the site at which the services are received, or their utilization. As such, it represents a continuum—from plans that, for example, do no more than require prior authorization of inpatient stays, to the staff model HMO that employs its doctors and assumes risk for delivering a comprehensive benefit package. Ideally managed care should not simply seek to reduce costs; rather it should strive to maximize value, which includes a concern with quality and access. (Fox 1990, 1)

The following characteristics are inherent in most definitions of managed care:

contracts with selected physicians and hospitals that furnish a comprehensive set of health care services to enrolled members, usually for a predetermined monthly premium;

utilization and quality controls that contracting providers agree to accept;

financial incentives for patients to use the providers and facilities associated with the plan;

the assumption of some financial risk by physicians, thus fundamentally altering their role from serving as agent for the patient's welfare to balancing the patient's needs against the need for cost control (Iglehart 1992a, 742).

Thus, the term *managed care* is used to refer to almost any alternative to traditional fee-for-service arrangements. It includes not only fee-for-service indemnity plans with minimal controls over utilization and costs but also highly organized systems that alter reimbursement mechanisms and control both the delivery system and provider behavior (see table I.1). As Hornbrook and Goodman pointed out, "managed care has come to denote a confusing variety of structures and strategies to improve the performance of the health care system; these range from reimbursement incentives to alternative delivery systems to detailed protocols guiding physician behavior" (Hornbrook and Goodman 1991, 107).

Most organizations that provide managed care are called either health maintenance organizations (HMOs) or preferred provider organizations (PPOs). The variations that exist within these categories reflect the rapid evolution of the organization and financing of health services in the United States (Iglehart 1992a). We will describe these in greater detail in chapter 1, below. Because managed care plans, such as PPOs and HMOs, integrate the delivery and financing of health care and have incentives that encourage providers to be more efficient, the growth of these plans could restrain inflation in health care costs and produce demonstrable savings. These systems are also more likely to have quality-assurance mechanisms. As more people enroll in these plans, price competition could force fee-for-service providers to become more efficient (Rosko and Broyles 1988).

Support for this approach is growing among major employers and among the managers of American business firms. A recent health policy article in *Fortune* (Faltermayer 1992) advocated a model that would require every American to enroll in an HMO or a similar managed care plan. This would be combined with outcomes research (to determine which medical procedures work best and which are wasteful) and continuous quality improvement (to enhance the quality of care and to make it more uniform throughout the U.S. health care system). These ideas are primarily based on the writings of Stanford economist Alain Enthoven, one of the originators of the concept of "managed competition," who views managed care as the only practical solution to the soaring cost of medical care (Enthoven 1981; Enthoven and Kronick 1991). Recently, the American Medical Association has accepted the legitimacy and benefits of managed care (Iglehart 1992a).

There is growing concern, however, that managed care will emphasize cost controls at the expense of access to care and that the care provided will be impersonal and unresponsive to people's needs. Consumers fear that their choice of physicians and hospitals will be greatly curtailed, and

Table I.1. The Managed Care Continuum

	Managed Care Plans						
	"Pure" Indemnity	Modified Indemnity	PPO	Open-ended HMO*	EPO	IPA HMO	"Pure" HMO
Utilization review	No utilization review →	Preadmission certification — Concurrent review — Second surgical opinion →	Management information system — Physician profiling →			Formal peer review →	Informal peer review — Protocols
Provider panel	No provider selection →		Selected providers →				Staff providers
Consumer choice of provider	Total freedom of choice →		Incentives to limit choice →		Lock-in →		
Benefit structure	Varied coverage — Deductibles, coinsurance — Routine preventive care uncovered →		Waives deductibles — Reduces coinsurance →			Comprehensive coverage including preventive care — Limited copayments	
Provider payment	Fee-for-service payment →					Withholds capitation →	Salary
Rating method	Experience rated →					Community rated →	
Practice setting	Independent practice →						Group practice

Source: Adapted from Hale and Hunter 1988, p. 13.

Abbreviations: PPO, preferred provider organizations; HMO, health maintenance organization; EPO, exclusive provider organization; IPA, independent practice association.

*An open-ended HMO is a hybrid plan that takes characteristics from both ends of the spectrum.

many physicians fear that managed care will restrict their medical decisions and their professional autonomy and lower the quality of care (Iglehart 1992a).

These concerns have heightened the need for better information on the performance of managed care. Much of the research that has been done on managed care has focused on its potential to contain costs (Wallack 1991), and several recent articles and books have dealt extensively with this issue (Rosko and Broyles 1988; Davis et al. 1990; Rice 1992; Iglehart 1992a). Considerable knowledge also exists regarding the quality of care provided by certain types of managed care organizations, particularly HMOs (Cunningham and Williamson 1980; Luft and Morrison 1991). Though cost containment and quality are of crucial importance, they are not the focus of this book. The potential of managed care to contain costs has dominated policy discussions while other major issues have been relatively ignored. Whether managed care will improve access and patient satisfaction are equally important concerns and have tended to be neglected in the current policy debates. The other critical question is the extent to which managed care can attract and retain qualified physicians. Acceptance by physicians may be more of a limiting factor to the expansion of managed care than any of the other issues.

During the early years of health plan development in the United States, many questions could be examined only on the basis of assumptions and personal experience (Darsky, Sinai, and Axelrod 1958; Greenlick, Freeborn, and Pope 1988). But today questions related to health services can be addressed more scientifically. Unsupported assumptions about many issues are no longer tenable because there are laboratories in which these assumptions can be tested. This situation provides the opportunity for basing health policy on a firm foundation of factual knowledge. Too seldom do health policy discussions take into account the experiences and research findings from existing health care laboratories.

The laboratories of health services are to be found throughout the United States. They consist of those alternative delivery systems that go beyond the patterns of traditional plans in covering more people or in providing more (and better) services at equal or lower costs. They are the systems that have broken new ground in financing and organizing services and that serve as models for newly emerging systems. Studying these systems can suggest ways to enhance existing arrangements and can provide the factual basis for improving the performance of health care systems. They can be viewed as demonstrations of what may be implemented as national health policy in the future (Luft and Morrison 1991).

In this book we focus primarily on the prepaid group practice HMO model of managed care, both in discussing the research literature and in reporting the results of our studies. This model is the most highly organized form of managed care in the United States and is the prototype for managed care. Although we discuss (in chapter 1) various hybrid models—such as independent practice associations (IPAs) and PPOs—that combine aspects of fee-for-service and of managed care, we make no attempt to compare these with the group practice model except by way of describing the respective underlying organizational concepts. To attempt to do more—for example, to compare physician or patient satisfaction across models—would inevitably prove futile, since empirical data comparable to what we have on HMOs are simply not available for these other organizations.

Nor do we compare the group practice managed care system in the United States with health care systems in other countries. To do so without taking into account the myriad historical, cultural, and social factors that influence the relative success or failure of such systems within their respective national contexts would make the validity or usefulness of such comparisons questionable. Certain statistical comparisons, of course, are easy enough to make—for example, that the United States spends a greater proportion of its gross domestic product on health care than does any other industrialized nation, that health services in other industrialized countries tend to be distributed more effectively throughout the population, or that Americans complain about their health care system more than do the citizens of other countries (Blendon 1989; Cockerham 1992; Kindig and Sullivan 1992). To render such comparisons meaningful, however, is far more complex. Rather than attempt such an undertaking, therefore, we have chosen to present as complete a description as possible of one managed care organization, the largest of its kind in the world, in the hope that those who undertake similar analyses of other models, either within the United States or abroad, will have a clearer understanding of the issues involved and of the extent to which such models are in fact comparable.

The primary audiences for this book are federal, state, and local policy makers, legislators, planners, health plan managers, and health professionals, and consumers and others who are interested in this topic but do not have specialized knowledge about managed care. The book could also serve as a supplementary text and an introduction to managed care for graduate students in public health, health services management and policy, the health professions, and the social sciences. Finally, there is growing international interest in managed care, and the book could serve as an introduction to the topic for a variety of international audiences.

Why This Book?

This book aims to contribute to a growing body of research and policy studies on managed health care. Its overall aim is to provide information to improve the delivery of health services and to contribute to the national debate about how best to organize health care. We hope to provide a balanced appraisal of the advantages and disadvantages of the prepaid group practice HMO model of managed care so that consumers and policy makers can make more informed decisions. In particular, we want to fill gaps in current knowledge about the likelihood of people's joining this form of managed care, people's access to services in such managed care settings, and the likelihood that patients and physicians will accept this form of managed care. The success of managed care as a national strategy would be seriously undermined if only a limited number of consumers and physicians would participate in this most integrated model of managed care, or if this form of care reduced costs at the expense of access and patient satisfaction.

Specifically, this book first examines a set of questions about patients and consumers. These include (1) Why do people choose the prepaid group practice HMO model of managed care in preference to traditional plans, and how do enrollees in this type of managed care system differ from persons who join traditional fee-for-service plans? (2) How do members' perceived needs for care relate to their actual use of services, and what problems do they have in accessing and using care? (3) How do members evaluate their experiences with this form of managed care, particularly with respect to access, costs, and the quality of care? (4) Why do members terminate their membership, and to what extent is the decision to leave a result of dissatisfaction?

A second set of questions focuses on physicians and their views of the advantages and disadvantages of the prepaid group practice HMO model of managed care. The specific issues addressed include (1) Why do physicians choose this form of practice? (2) To what extent do physicians feel that professional autonomy and the ability to provide good medical care are compromised in this kind of setting? (3) What are the major sources of job satisfaction and dissatisfaction among physicians who practice in this kind of setting? and (4) How do physicians view access, quality, and other aspects of care in this setting?

Each of these issues deals with an important dimension of managed care, whatever its specific form. If managed care plans are to be successful and viable as a policy option, they must be able to attract and retain members. To a large degree, this depends on providing reasonable levels of access at reasonable costs. The quality and continuity of care must also be acceptable to patients. In addition, consumers often evaluate health services on the basis of the quality of interactions with physicians and other staff members, and these day-to-day interactions may be more important than the purely technical aspects of care.

At the same time, HMO managed care systems must be able to recruit qualified physicians and other health professionals and motivate them to achieve high levels of performance. To do so, managed care must provide a satisfying work environment, as well as adequate financial rewards. High levels of dissatisfaction can lower performance and increase turnover among physicians and other health care workers. Turnover and poor performance are costly to organizations and adversely affect the quality and continuity of care for patients (Lichtenstein 1984b). Thus, it is important to study physician satisfaction because it can play a major role in organizational effectiveness and the long-range viability of managed care. The potential of the HMO model of managed care as a solution to the health care crisis, and the stability of the HMO as a practice setting, both depend on maintaining reasonable levels of satisfaction for both patients and health care providers.

The Setting for This Book

The setting (and laboratory) for this work is Kaiser Permanente, Northwest Region (KPNW), a federally qualified prepaid group practice HMO serving more than 375,000 members in the greater Portland, Oregon, and Vancouver, Washington, metropolitan area. KPNW provides comprehensive medical care for a fixed, prepaid fee with minimal copayments and deductibles. It is a nonprofit community service program. Unlike insurance plans that simply share in the cost of medical and hospital services, KPNW provides or arranges for medical and hospital care and assumes responsibility for both the quality and the cost of the care it provides. Five basic principles have shaped the organization of this system: voluntary enrollment; prepayment for comprehensive benefits on a service basis; preventive medical care; integrated, hospital-based health care facilities; and the provision of physician services through group medical practice.

KPNW evolved from industrial health care programs for shipyard workers in the Pacific Northwest during the late 1930s and 1940s and was opened to public enrollment in 1945. It is organized into three entities: the Kaiser Foundation Health Plan (a nonprofit health plan corporation that enrolls members, manages finances, and maintains membership records); Northwest Permanente (an independent professional corporation that provides medical care); and Kaiser Foundation Hospitals (a nonprofit and charitable hospital corporation that owns and operates two hospitals and seventeen medical offices in the Portland-Vancouver area). Physicians and managers share responsibility for significant policy, planning, and resource allocation decisions. Further details on KPNW's organizational structure and its operating characteristics are provided in subsequent chapters (also see Greenlick, Freeborn, and Pope 1988; Kaiser Permanente 1992).

Given the aims of this book, this setting is appropriate for a variety of reasons. First, the stability and maturity of KPNW allow us to examine various dimensions of managed care without having to be concerned about the confounding effects introduced in organizations undergoing major transitions. As Madison and Konrad (1988) point out, many health care organizations today are in transition and are moving from the traditional fee-for-service arrangements toward some form of managed care. KPNW has provided services in the Pacific Northwest for nearly half a century, making it one of the oldest regional HMOs and managed care systems in the United States.

Second, this setting provides large study populations of both patients and providers, thus affording opportunities for more detailed analyses than can be performed in many other settings.

Third, Kaiser Permanente (KP) is the prototypical prepaid group practice plan that provided the model for the HMO concept and for managed care. As a prepaid group practice HMO, KP has become the benchmark for other managed care plans. KP and similar large group practice HMOs have also been described as the most highly bureaucratic of the various types of practice arrangements (Wolinsky 1985). Concerns have been expressed about the potential negative impact of bureaucratization on patients and providers (see chapter 1), and Kaiser Permanente, Northwest Region, offers a relevant setting in which this issue can empirically be examined.

A fourth reason for using this setting is the availability of extensive high-quality empirical data collected over many years. The data sources include a community survey and surveys of KPNW members, patients, and physicians, as well as comprehensive medical records and KPNW membership files. These are described briefly in appropriate chapters in the book and are cited in the figures displaying the data. More details about the data sources and data collection methods are given in the Appendix, below. Most of the data sets have been developed by the authors and their colleagues at the Kaiser Permanente Center for Health Research (CHR). When figures are based on these data sets, the figure legends include the source of the data and the year in which the data were obtained. The time frames for the data presented vary for several reasons. Not only were the questions asked in some surveys not asked in others, but we chose for practical reasons to focus our analysis on a few surveys that asked relatively more of the questions pertinent to the subject of this book. Our findings from these analyses, however, are very consistent with similar or comparable data we have examined in others of our surveys over the years.

The CHR conducts a broad program of public-domain health care research using KPNW as its research setting. The CHR was established as a not-for-profit, professionally autonomous research institute that is organizationally a part of KPNW. The CHR also has an affiliation agreement with the Oregon Health Sciences University providing for collaboration and joint sponsorship of research and other activities. The CHR research program is supported primarily through grants and contracts from federal agencies, including the National Institutes of Health. The work of the investigators is peer reviewed and published in professional and scientific journals. CHR investigators decide on the research questions and are legally and ethically responsible for the conduct of the research (see Greenlick, Freeborn, and Pope 1988 for a more complete discussion of this issue).

The Plan of This Book

Chapter 1 provides a brief history of managed care and describes the major types of managed care. Chapter 2 focuses on why people choose alternative plans and the characteristics that differentiate people who choose the KPNW prepaid group practice plan from those who do not. Chapter 3 examines factors influencing access to and the use of services in KPNW, and the relationship between people's perceived need for care and their actual use of services. Chapter 4 deals with how consumers evaluate their experiences with the KPNW managed care system and their level of satisfaction with access, costs, and the quality of care and service. Chapter 5 focuses on physicians' views of the KPNW managed care system and on factors influencing physician satisfaction. In chapters 2 through 5, we provide a brief review of the key policy issues related to the topic under consideration. We then present our results and point out how they relate to the larger body of knowledge about managed care. Chapter 6 builds on but goes beyond the findings presented in the previous chapters to discuss managed care generally and the implications of managed care for national health policy.

Some see managed care as a panacea for health care, but for others it conjures up the worst nightmares of "bureaucratic medicine." However one feels about it, managed care in some form is likely to become the dominant form of medical care delivery, and we need to have a better understanding of its potential impact on both the patients and the providers of care. As a nation, we seem to be at a crucial juncture in our history: a time in which significant changes will occur in the way in which we organize and finance health services. We hope that this book will help inform the national debate on this issue and contribute to more rational and effective health policy.

The Rise of Managed Care

> Managed care is better than unmanaged care.
> —Ernest W. Saward, M.D.

Although some forms of managed care have existed for many years, most Americans have received care through traditional fee-for-service arrangements that allow patients to choose their own physician and physicians to practice with few constraints on their clinical decisions. Employer-sponsored health insurance has been the primary mechanism for financing medical care in the United States, and the choice of health insurance has been a private, voluntary matter. Although many policy makers, politicians, and third-party payers support managed care, it is not accepted as widely by the American public and the medical profession. Managed care places restrictions on both patients and physicians, and we have limited knowledge regarding the extent to which it will be accepted and the likelihood of its improving access to care and contributing to other hoped-for outcomes. In this chapter, we discuss some of the major issues and concerns about managed care, as well as the potential of managed care for solving the problems of the medical care system. We also describe the various forms of managed care and what we know about their performance. First, however, we need to provide some historical background on the organization and financing of health services in the United States and the development of managed care. The purpose is to help us understand why managed care has become the centerpiece of health care reform.

The Development of Managed Care

Where or when the concept of managed care originated is hard to say. In the United States the concept dates back to at least 1798, when Congress established the Marine Hospital Service, a system of hospitals with salaried medical staffs that provided prepaid services to merchant seamen. The more immediate predecessors in the United States were the nineteenth-century medical mutuals and "friendly societies" that were developed in Europe and in lands colonized by Europeans. In 1929, the physician Michael Shadid and the Farmers' Union in Beckham County, Oklahoma, established the Community Hospital Association of Elk City, generally acknowledged as the first full-scale prepaid medical cooperative in the United States (Luft 1981). The most significant and comprehensive approach to the concept of managed care can be traced to the series of reports issued by the Committee on the Costs of Medical Care (CCMC) between 1927 and 1932 (reprinted in CCMC 1972).

The CCMC recognized the many shortcomings of the traditional fee-for-service system and recommended a more organized approach. "The problem [the difficulty of providing high-quality medical care] will not solve itself through the operation of undirected economic forces. Some conscious redirection of medical activities is needed, and long-term planning with a clear vision of the objectives to be achieved" (Lee and Jones 1933, 127). The CCMC made a number of recommendations to improve the system of medical care delivery in the United States. Its first recommendation was, "Medical service, both preventive and therapeutic, should be furnished largely by organized groups of physicians, dentists, nurses, pharmacists, and other associated personnel. Such groups should be organized, preferably around a hospital, for rendering complete home, office, and hospital care. The form of organization should encourage the maintenance of high standards and the development or preservation of a personal relation between patient and physician" (CCMC 1972, 109).

The committee felt that this arrangement not only would result in better use of specialists and improvements in quality but also would be more convenient and economical for the patient. The committee also urged that the costs of medical care be met on a group prepayment basis and recommended required health insurance for low-income groups. Finally, it called for the development of improved mechanisms for coordinating and evaluating preventive and curative medical services to eliminate unneeded services and to create new and additional services if required (CCMC 1972).

This farsighted plan for "managed care" was not to be. The only examples of managed care at that time were the few pioneer prepaid group practice plans, and these covered a very small segment of the population. Eventually, research would provide data on the performance of a number of these early versions of managed care, but this information was not available to the CCMC (Shapiro 1984). Fee-for-service practice was to remain the predominant form of medical practice during this period; the recommendations of the CCMC were largely ignored. Organized medicine was opposed to the CCMC's recommendations and was able to control the content of medical care and the way in which medical care was organized and financed (Starr 1982).

During World War II health insurance was promoted as a fringe benefit of employment in the United States, and this greatly stimulated the growth of private health insurance (Knickman and Thorpe 1990). Existing health insurance strongly emphasized inpatient coverage; and not surprisingly, the general hospital became the dominant institution. The community general hospital was about the only organized component of the medical care system and was to become the center for the expansion of medical technology (Somers and Somers 1961). Most physicians, however, practiced alone or in small fee-for-service groups. The hospital was the physician's "workshop," but physicians were primarily independent contractors who were only loosely affiliated with hospitals or other medical organizations. Financing was mainly provided by nonprofit insurance plans such as Blue Cross and Blue Shield, or by for-profit commercial insurance plans. These agencies had little influence or control over the organization of medical care; they mainly processed claims and reimbursed hospitals and physicians.

The passage of legislation establishing Medicare and Medicaid in 1965 provided increased public financing for health services and enhanced access for elderly persons and the poor (Davis 1991). However, these programs were specifically required not to interfere with the private practice of medicine or to infringe upon professional autonomy. The preamble to the Medicare law expressly prohibits any federal "supervision or control over the practice of medicine or the manner in which medical services are provided." Without this provision, opposition by organized medicine and the private health insurance industry probably would have prevented the passage of the legislation. Hospital planning councils (and later, local health systems agencies) were set up and supported by the federal government in the 1960s and 1970s, but these agencies had little power and were dominated by the providers of care. These agencies had limited authority (and resources) with which to manage or control the complex array of financing institutions, hospitals, physicians, and other providers of care (Thorpe 1990). Various attempts at regulation, such as requirements for certificates of need, and hospital rate setting, were attempted in the 1970s and 1980s, but these were cost-containment strategies and were not, strictly speaking, "managed care" (Rice 1992).

The passage by Congress of the Health Maintenance Organization

Act (Public Law 93-222) in 1973 was an endorsement of fundamental change in the nation's system of health care delivery. This legislation greatly stimulated the growth of health maintenance organizations. HMOs were a major departure from conventional health insurance, the dominant method for financing medical care in the United States at this time. HMOs assume responsibility for providing medical care to a defined population that has enrolled voluntarily. In addition, HMOs integrate financing and service delivery in a single organization and accept responsibility for the quality of care they provide. They also assume responsibility for providing the needed services within a fixed budget and thus avoid unpredictable cost overruns—a feature that is very appealing to policy makers (Luft and Morrison 1991).

Paul Ellwood was the first to refer to this form of delivery system as a "health maintenance organization." His use of the term was part of a political strategy to obtain the Nixon administration's support and congressional approval for prepaid medical care as an alternative to traditional fee-for-service practice. The Nixon administration endorsed HMOs as the new national health strategy in 1971 and pressed Congress to enact laws to encourage HMO development through planning grants and loans. The underlying reason for this support of the growth of HMOs was the belief that HMOs would stimulate competition among alternative health plans and slow the rate of increase in health care expenditures. This approach was compatible with the ideology of the Nixon administration, which held that competition among health plans would enhance efficiency as well as consumer choice. The passage of the Health Maintenance Organization Act of 1973 provided the initial stimulus for the growth of HMOs in the middle and late 1970s (Davis et al. 1990).

The federal government promoted HMOs as its primary strategy to bring about an efficient and equitable medical care system. HMOs were the major examples of managed care in the 1970s, and the large prepaid group practice HMOs often combined the major elements of care (including the financing, the facilities and hospitals, and the medical personnel) under one management structure. The government's goal was to have one thousand HMOs by 1980, with the expectation that more than 90 percent of U.S. citizens would have access to an alternative form of health care delivery. This goal was not achieved, although enrollment in HMOs grew more than tenfold between 1970 and 1990 (Welch, Hillman, and Pauly 1990; Wallack 1991; Iglehart 1992a). In the past two decades, managed care has become a major force in altering the form of health care delivery in the United States. Much of managed care incorporates the principles of HMOs; for instance, most managed care organizations serve defined populations, manage patient treatment, use a select group of physicians and hospitals, and place the providers at financial risk.

Costs and cost containment dominated health policy during the 1980s. The Reagan administration's view was that the free market and competition would solve the problems of the health care system, particularly if government's role could be reduced to a minimum (Starr 1982). The Reagan administration cut public health services and reduced public financing for personal health services for the poor. The health care regulatory system was seen as wasteful and inefficient, and a major goal of the Reagan administration was to replace regulation with market competition. Regulatory approaches such as health systems agencies (which had overseen planning and regulation at local levels) were phased out. The strategies that gained acceptance included increased patient cost sharing (e.g., copayments and deductibles), requirements for second opinions and preadmission certification for certain types of cases, and expansions in utilization management generally (Rice 1992).

Policy makers in the 1980s also focused on cost-containment strategies that targeted providers. The establishment of the Prospective Payment System (PPS) using Diagnosis-Related Groups (DRGs) for paying hospitals is the most important example. This system provides fixed amounts of dollars for specific hospital admissions, instead of reimbursing providers for all "usual, customary, and reasonable" services (Luft and Morrison 1991). It has resulted in a decline in hospital admissions and reduced the length of hospital stays for Medicare patients. From a cost standpoint, DRGs seem to have been successful (Rice 1992). In 1989, Congress approved major changes in Medicare physician payment. Both DRGs and the legislation reforming physician payments apply only to Medicare. They focus on reimbursement and changing the payment system—not on restructuring the way in which health services are organized. Many analysts and policy makers point out that service delivery mechanisms must also be changed, and most proposals to reform the U.S. health care system, including the recent Clinton administration proposal, emphasize managed care.

Traditional arrangements that permit patients to choose their own physicians and to get reimbursed for all or part of whatever physicians and hospitals charge are steadily decreasing. More and more patients and providers are now involved in plans that place some restrictions on both patients and providers. By 1990, the majority of employees nationwide were enrolled in some form of managed care (Iglehart 1992a). However, many people are still in fee-for-service indemnity plans that allow them to choose any physician they want and be reimbursed a set percentage of the resulting bill. Most so-called managed care plans monitor utilization (some also provide case management for high-cost patients), but they do not fundamentally change the way in which medical care is paid for or delivered.

The Larger Medical Care Context

The phenomenon of managed care must be viewed in the larger context of the bureaucratization of medicine in general. The 1970s and 1980s also saw an increase in the number of large, multiple-hospital systems operated by powerful corporate management (Starr 1982). Although nonprofit hospitals still predominate, the for-profit chains such as the Hospital Corporation of America and Humana account for most of the recent growth in multiple-hospital systems. This represents a fundamental change in the U.S. medical care system. Traditionally, the pattern has been freestanding general hospitals governed by their own local boards, administrators, and medical staffs. According to sociologist Paul Starr, "Corporations have begun to integrate a hitherto decentralized hospital system, enter a variety of other health care businesses, and consolidate ownership and control in what may eventually become an industry dominated by huge health care conglomerates" (Starr 1982, 428).

The concentration of power may erode professional autonomy, further aggravate inequalities in access to health care, and greatly reduce public accountability and participation (Starr 1982; Navarro 1988). The ability of health professionals and consumers to control medical care organizations has diminished, while the power of managers and corporate control has increased. Professional managers now have more control over decisions that affect both the nature and the operation of health care institutions (Greenlick 1989). In addition, many medical leaders are concerned that a business ethos will become dominant among medical care providers and institutions. Nonprofit organizations have traditionally dominated the health care sector (Gray 1986), and the culture of medicine has emphasized the ideals of professionalism and service to the patient. Arnold Relman, a physician and a distinguished former editor of the *New England Journal of Medicine,* argued that physicians are increasingly becoming businessmen and that medicine is in danger of losing its ethical way. He felt that if physicians continue to be lured by entrepreneurial values, they will lose the public trust and their opportunity to reform medical practice in positive ways (Relman 1992a).

Medicine's adoption of market values and the trend toward corporate medicine are dangerous for patients and for society as a whole, according to Relman. He stated:

> If most of our physicians become entrepreneurs and most of our hospitals and health-care facilities become businesses, paying patients will get more care than they need and poor patients will get less. In a commercialized system the cost of health care will continue to escalate and yet we will not be assured of getting the kind of care we really need. In such a system, we will no longer be able to trust our physicians, because the bond of fiduciary responsibility will have been broken. (Relman 1992a, 106)

A number of analysts, however, contend that medicine in the United States has always been dominated by market values and that physicians have traditionally been private entrepreneurs who sell their services on a for-profit basis. Princeton economist Uwe Reinhardt, for example, eloquently argued that physicians are no different from other purveyors of goods and services. In a series of published letters between Reinhardt and Relman, Reinhardt suggested that the more fundamental question is one of social values—namely, whether as a nation we want to continue to treat health care as a consumer good or whether we should treat it as a community service to be distributed on the basis of medical need (Relman and Reinhardt 1986).

Increasingly, physicians are being pressured to affiliate with some type of organization to ensure themselves of a practice and an adequate income. These changes threaten professional autonomy and may lead to a reduction in physicians' control over professional decisions. A basic shift may be under way that will decrease collegial control among physicians and substitute corporate control (Madison and Konrad 1988). Starr pointed out:

> The failure to rationalize medical services under public control meant that sooner or later they would be rationalized under private control. Instead of public regulation, there will be private regulation, and instead of public planning, there will be corporate planning. Instead of public financing for prepaid plans that might be managed by the subscribers' chosen representatives, there will be corporate financing for private plans controlled by conglomerates whose interests will be determined by the rate of return on investments. That is the future toward which American medicine now seems to be headed. (Starr 1982, 449)

These trends and shifts in power and control have led to growing fears that financial objectives will dominate our medical institutions at the expense of patients' needs. Patients who cannot pay may be increasingly turned away or referred to already overburdened public hospitals. As the health care system becomes increasingly organized and bureaucratic, relationships may become more segmented and impersonal, with physicians acting primarily as organizational officials or bureaucrats. As the system's gatekeepers, physicians may give greater priority to organizational demands and may sacrifice the quality of patient care (Starr 1982; Mechanic 1986). The common view is that increased bureaucratization is equivalent to dehumanization.

Many observers, however, have pointed out that more highly organized systems offer great promise for enhancing quality as well as efficiency (Shortell and Kaluzny 1988). Some research, for example, suggests that physicians perform better in settings where there are specific, objective rules concerning admission to the staff and requirements for continued membership in the staff (Smith and Kaluzny 1986). Research also suggests that hospital and medical staff members perform better when administrators and chiefs of staff maintain operating statistics to monitor performance, and that medical staffs perform better when they are more formally organized (Shortell 1991). That is to say, increased organization can enhance both effectiveness and operating efficiency.

The most significant aspect of increased organization is its capacity for facilitating rational planning and coordination to achieve desired goals. Thus, planning for and consciously dealing with troublesome but fundamental aspects of medical care (such as the supply and use of medical personnel, access to care, the quality and cost of care, patient satisfaction, and physician morale) can lead to improved performance. In contrast to unrestrained market forces, these more deliberate and planned processes can result in a more efficient application of human ingenuity to problems in providing medical care. The challenge is to design systems of care that enhance human values and maintain professional autonomy while taking advantage of advances in knowledge and technology and the benefits of large-scale organization.

Although many U.S. citizens are still covered by conventional fee-for-service plans, an increasing number are enrolling in managed care plans such as health maintenance organizations and preferred provider organizations. Most organizations that provide managed care are either HMOs or PPOs, and these plans constitute the most highly organized systems in the United States (although there is some variation within each of these forms of managed care). Many observers feel that HMOs and PPOs offer the most promise in terms of controlling costs without compromising quality, and these systems are receiving the most attention as policy options. In the following sections, we describe the characteristics of these forms of managed care and discuss some of their advantages and disadvantages.

Health Maintenance Organizations

HMOs are the most highly structured and organized systems of care in the private sector. Although there are several forms of HMO, they all have the following characteristics (Luft 1981, 2):

The HMO assumes a contractual responsibility to provide or to ensure the delivery of a stated range of health services. This includes at least ambulatory care and inpatient services.

The HMO provides services to a population defined by enrollment in the plan.

Enrollment is voluntary.

The subscriber pays a fixed annual or monthly payment (premium) that is independent of the use of services.

The HMO assumes at least part of the financial risk in the provision of services.

Although historically HMO enrollment has been voluntary, this is changing rapidly. Many HMOs are offering special incentives (e.g., multiple-year contracts at discounted premiums) to employers that select them as sole carrier. HMOs generally have more benefits and better coverage than do traditional indemnity insurance and PPO plans (Hale and Hunter 1988; Luft and Morrison 1991). HMO members are guaranteed access to all basic health services with only limited additional out-of-pocket expenses, such as modest copayments for office visits. Members are required to use participating physicians and are enrolled for specified time periods. In most HMOs, primary care physicians are expected to act as gatekeepers. That is to say, they are to serve as the basic point of entry for HMO members, and the mechanism by which members are referred to specialists. This is designed to promote more appropriate use of specialists and other services. It also places more constraints on patients than do traditional fee-for-service plans and PPOs (Iglehart 1992a).

Enrollment in HMOs increased more than tenfold between 1970 and 1991—from 3.6 million persons to more than 37 million. However, current HMO enrollees represent only 14 percent of all U.S. citizens and less than 25 percent of those with private health insurance (Welch 1987; Wallack 1991; Porter and Ball 1992).

There are four basic HMO models—the group model, the staff model, the network model, and the independent practice association (see fig. 1.1). These can be differentiated on the basis of how physician services are organized and how physicians are paid (Davis et al. 1990; Hornbrook and Goodman 1991).

The group-model HMO usually provides the hospitals and other physical facilities and employs the nonphysician clinical personnel. It also provides the administrative support staff. The HMO contracts with one large (professionally autonomous) multiple-specialty medical group practice for physician services. The HMO pays the medical group a monthly amount per member to provide medical services. Payment to the individual physician is determined by the medical group, and the physicians are paid the equivalent of a salary (instead of a fee for every procedure performed). The physicians usually restrict their practices to HMO members only, and are at risk financially for the services they provide (Davis et al. 1990). In 1991, approximately 27 percent of all HMO members (9,654,880 persons) were in group-model HMOs (fig. 1.1).

In staff-model HMOs, the HMO hires the physicians, who are paid a salary to provide health services. Thus, the physicians are employees of the HMO and work only for the HMO. They are generally not at risk financially for the services they provide. The HMO is still at risk, however. Unlike their counterparts in the group model, physicians in the staff model are not part of autonomous and independent medical groups, but they still practice primarily in multispecialty groups. Approximately 8 percent of all HMO members in 1991 were in staff-model HMOs.

Network-model HMOs differ from group-model HMOs in several ways. A network-model HMO contracts with more than one physician group, and the physician groups provide the facilities and employ the nonphysician personnel. Each physician group in the network receives a capitation payment (a monthly amount per member) for the members who obtain care from that group. Most such physician groups also provide care to fee-for-service patients. Eleven percent of all HMO members were enrolled in network HMOs in 1991.

Staff-, group-, and network-model HMOs are often referred to as prepaid group practices (PGPs). The combination of multiple-specialty group practice and capitation payment is thought to enhance economies of scale, and peer review. As pointed out by Hornbrook and Goodman, "capitation payment is an indirect financial incentive that shifts the

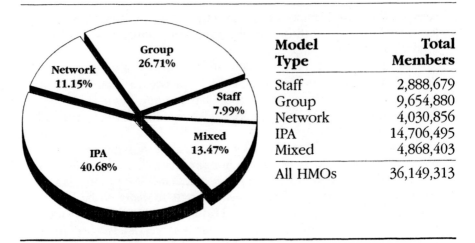

Model Type	Total Members
Staff	2,888,679
Group	9,654,880
Network	4,030,856
IPA	14,706,495
Mixed	4,868,403
All HMOs	36,149,313

Fig. 1.1. HMO enrollment by model type as of January 1, 1992.
Source: Data from Porter and Ball 1992, 4.

financial risk of caring for an individual enrollee entirely to the health plan (HMO) and stimulates establishment of a prospective budgeting system for managing access and care" (Hornbrook and Goodman 1991, 109). The inherent advantages of medical practice in more organized settings are considerably enhanced, it can be argued, when combined with a capitation reimbursement arrangement. For a given budgetary period, capitation results in a fixed pool of money that is available for meeting the costs of providing care. As a result, providers tend to become more cost conscious, and administrative controls develop to achieve cost-effective routines of care through such means as efficiency in production of services, more prudent use of services, a different combination or mix of services, practice guidelines, or similar mechanisms.

The last HMO model is the independent practice association, the fastest-growing and dominant form of HMO. In this arrangement, the HMO uses a percentage of the time of many independent practitioners to provide care to its subscribers. Physicians continue to practice in their own offices but agree to treat patients enrolled in the HMO. The HMO contracts with a number of independent physicians, who generally are paid on a fee-for-service basis (Davis et al. 1990). However, capitation contracts are becoming more common, and in a number of cases IPA primary care physicians are directly responsible for paying some portion of referral costs out of their capitation. Approximately 41 percent of all HMO members were in IPAs in 1992.

IPAs permit physicians to remain in independent practice but also accept risk for a defined population via contractual arrangements. In an IPA, physicians see both HMO patients and non-HMO patients. Most IPA-model HMOs reimburse participating physicians according to agreed-upon fee schedules. IPAs tend to have a greater number of participating physicians than do group-model HMOs. Thus, IPA members have more options and a wider choice of physicians than do members of PGPs (Rosko and Broyles 1988; Davis et al. 1990). IPA participating physicians have individual offices dispersed throughout the community, an arrangement that limits interaction with colleagues and peer review but that may be more convenient for patients. Participating physicians may be less committed to the HMO form of practice or to HMO patients, since the physicians may receive only a small portion of their income from the HMO. Nevertheless, IPAs are growing three times faster than group-model HMOs and may dominate the HMO industry in the future (Welch 1987; Porter and Ball 1992).

Most studies of HMO performance have compared fee-for-service plans with the large, well-established, prepaid group practice HMOs and have various methodological shortcomings (Rosko and Broyles 1988). The results of these studies have been summarized in a number of review articles and books (Weinerman 1964; Donabedian 1969; Greenlick 1972; Hetherington, Hopkins, and Roemer 1975; Luft 1980; Luft 1981; Rosko and Broyles 1988; Davis et al. 1990). As we might expect, much of the research has dealt with costs, the area of most concern to policy makers.

In fee-for-service practice, physician income is positively related to the number of services provided. The incentives are reversed in HMOs, where profitability is related to reductions in the volume of services provided. Accordingly, costs per member are expected to be lower in HMOs than in traditional plans. In general, research supports this assumption and indicates that group- and staff-model HMOs can take care of a population at lower cost than can traditional insurance plans. The average costs per member are 10–40 percent lower in HMOs than in fee-for-service plans, and members' out-of-pocket costs are also lower (Luft 1981; Manning et al. 1984; Iglehart 1992a; Staines 1993). Most of the cost savings achieved by HMOs are due to decreased hospital utilization, primarily reductions in admission rates rather than reductions in length of stay (Luft 1978; Luft 1981; Rosko and Broyles 1988; Davis et al. 1990). The RAND study, a randomized controlled trial of health insurance, concluded that these savings are primarily due to the less hospital-intensive style of medicine practiced in HMOs (Manning et al. 1984). IPAs have also reduced their rates of hospital use in recent years, and many IPAs now have utilization rates comparable to those of group-model HMOs. More and more, IPA physicians are subject to formal utilization review mechanisms and to financial incentives to control costs (Davis et al. 1990).

Although HMOs have been found to provide care at lower cost, critics suggest that they may do so by reducing necessary services and lowering the quality of care (Wolinsky 1980). This concern has led to many studies comparing the quality of care in HMOs with that in fee-for-service practice (Cunningham and Williamson 1980; Donabedian 1985; Rosko and Broyles 1988). Existing research indicates that the technical quality of care in large group- and staff-model HMOs is equivalent to or better than that provided in fee-for-service plans (Luft 1981; Ware et al. 1986; Luft 1988; Greenlick, Freeborn, and Pope 1988). Though this seems to be true of large, mature, and established staff- and group-model HMOs, evidence is lacking on whether it holds for newer HMOs, IPAs, or the other forms of HMOs (Luft and Morrison 1991).

Quality has been measured by examining the characteristics of providers (e.g., place and type of medical training, specialty certification, availability of equipment, and accreditation status), and by process evaluations, which consist of reviews (medical audits) of the actions of physicians and other providers (Donabedian 1969; Luft 1981; Rosko and Broyles 1988). Relatively few studies have compared the outcomes of care in alternative plans, but those that have done so have consistently found that the outcomes of care in HMOs are as good as or better than the outcomes of fee-for-service practice (Shapiro, Weiner, and Densen 1958; Donabedian 1969; Cunningham and Williamson 1980; Luft 1981; Ware et al. 1986; Luft and Morrison 1991). Research on the quality of care provided by IPAs is very limited, however (Welch 1987).

In light of the performance of HMOs over the past several decades, many observers think that HMOs constitute the most promising alternative for containing health care costs while also enhancing the quality of care. For example, Relman stated: "In my opinion, a greater reliance on group practice and more emphasis on medical insurance that prepays providers at a fixed annual rate offer the best chance of solving the economic problems of health care, because these arrangements put physicians in the most favorable position to act as prudent advocates for their patients, rather than as entrepreneurial vendors of services" (Relman 1992a, 106).

The past growth of HMOs also suggests that consumers have considered HMO services to be acceptable and to be competitive with regard to cost. Recently, however, growth has slowed, and competition from other types of plans has intensified (Hale and Hunter 1988). In particular, preferred provider organizations are growing rapidly and appear to offer many advantages to both consumers and providers (Davis et al. 1990; Hosek and Marquis 1990). In the final section of this chapter, we define PPOs and discuss some of the major advantages and disadvantages of this form of managed care.

Preferred Provider Organizations

A preferred provider organization is an "arrangement in which a group of health care providers agrees to deliver care on a fee-for-service basis to a defined group of patients at an agreed-upon set of charges" (Rosko and Broyles 1988, 328). PPOs have in common five characteristics:

a provider panel limited to a specific group of physicians and hospitals,
negotiated compensation arrangements,
controls over provider behavior and use of resources (utilization review),
consumer choice of provider combined with incentives to use PPO
    providers,
rapid settlement of provider claims.

PPOs were first developed during the 1980s and have grown rapidly. The number of households enrolled in PPOs was 1.3 million in 1984; by 1989, it had increased to more than 18 million (Rice 1992; Iglehart 1992a). A PPO plan is similar to a traditional indemnity plan in that the cost of covered services is usually paid by the insurance plan after the services have been used. PPOs differ from traditional fee-for-service plans in two ways: the insurer plays a greater role in negotiating payment rates or choosing providers on the basis of lower expected costs; and physicians and hospitals are informed in advance that they must be subject to strong controls over use of services (Davis et al. 1990).

PPOs provide physician and hospital services at a discount, usually 10–20 percent. A PPO encourages its members to choose physicians from its roster by setting reduced copayments or deductibles for those physicians' services. However, the plan does not usually link a patient with a primary care physician who serves as a gatekeeper. In most PPOs, patients can seek care directly from specialists. Although PPOs do allow members to see physicians not on the roster, those who do so incur greater out-of-pocket expenses because higher copayments and deductibles are imposed.

PPOs appear to offer something for everybody involved: for employers, lower costs; for members, low out-of-pocket expenses, freedom of choice, and fee-for-service payment; and for providers, high patient volume. Although many employers think that PPOs are cost effective, no strong empirical evidence supports these assumptions (Davis et al. 1990). Little is known about the use of PPO benefits or about the actual cost savings achieved by PPOs (Rosko and Broyles 1988). The few studies that exist suggest that PPOs have not been successful in containing costs and that their activity may have resulted in higher utilization and costs (Rice 1992). Physicians in PPOs are still paid on a fee-for-service basis. All that a physician has to do to offset the financial effect of a PPO's discounts is to increase the intensity of services, generating more billings. PPOs have few incentives for cost-conscious medical practice, and PPO physicians are not at financial risk for services provided. PPO members have a financial incentive to use preferred providers, but they may also use providers outside the PPO, thus eroding the financial advantages of a PPO. PPOs, therefore, may not affect the overall inflation in medical care prices. PPOs are likely to continue to grow, but this raises several significant concerns for social policy. The growth of PPOs may further decrease access to care for poor people and persons without health insurance. Hospitals and physicians cannot take the chance of passing bad debts on to PPO patients. Second, overattention to cost may result in inadequate attention to quality differences among providers. Lower-cost providers may offer inferior care. Finally, favorable treatment of lower-cost providers and hospitals may lead to increased financial difficulties for teaching hospitals, further decreasing support for and the quality of graduate medical education and medical research (Davis et al. 1990).

Few studies have been conducted on patient or physician satisfaction with PPOs, but their growth suggests that PPOs are acceptable to both groups. PPOs retain many of the features of conventional plans, such as choice of providers, independent practice of medicine, and fee-for-service payment—features that may in many cases make them more attractive than HMOs (Hosek and Marquis 1990). However, no rigorous research has been conducted on the quality of care provided by PPOs (Davis et al. 1990; Luft and Morrison 1991). With increasing numbers of older patients and patients with chronic disease and disabilities, fragmentation of service is likely to remain a problem. PPOs have little to offer in terms of improving the coordination and continuity of care. The continuity of care is not likely to be enhanced, since the structure of medical practice remains unchanged and patients may or may not have a regular primary care provider. PPO physicians are community practitioners who practice alone or in fee-for-service groups. This situation provides little opportunity for ongoing peer review or formal quality-assurance mechanisms. Most PPO providers do not practice in a common location or share medical records with other providers. Thus, they are not likely to know a great deal about the medical care and treatment provided to their patients by other PPO physicians or by providers outside of the PPO. Finally, PPOs are not eligible for federal qualification as HMOs are, so there is no independent check on the financial soundness or quality of care of the PPO plan (Davis et al. 1990). It should be noted that, with increasing competition, many HMOs, at the request of employers, are also electing not to seek federal qualification.

As we have seen, most legislative proposals for dealing with the health care crisis include a strong role for managed care. However, there is still considerable controversy about the acceptability and cost-effectiveness of managed care and about whether it can be implemented nationwide. Although some forms of managed care have been shown to be less costly than conventional plans, the future success of managed care as a national strategy will depend on a number of factors in addition to cost containment. Up to this point, managed care plans have competed on the basis of price and reputation, but not on the basis of demonstrated and documented quality of care. In addition, managed care plans will have to demonstrate that they can attract and retain members and do a better job than traditional plans in terms of providing access to and continuity of care. They will also have to provide reasonable levels of satisfaction for both consumers and providers. These are the basic issues examined in the subsequent chapters of this book.

2

Choosing a Managed Care Plan

> Life is the art of drawing sufficient conclusions
> from insufficient premises.
> —Samuel Butler

Most major sectors of American society now agree that everyone has a right to health care. The major unsettled issues have to do with how access to care is going to be assured for everyone, how much and what kind of care each person is entitled to have, and how such care is going to be financed. It is clear that access will be through the mechanism of insurance, not through the creation of a national health service, as in Great Britain, and that most people are going to have some kind of choice. Freedom of choice is a basic American value. Freedom of choice in health care has traditionally meant choice among fee-for-service physicians and, to a lesser extent, among hospitals. This is congruent with the norms and ethics of medicine and hence has been strongly supported by the profession as well as by society through laws that recognize the special or privileged nature of the physician-patient relationship.

Whereas freedom of choice of physician remains a central value in health care, people have increasingly selected alternatives to the traditional fee-for-service system—alternatives that restrict or limit their choice of physicians. It seems increasingly likely that the first health care choice people will make in the future is what managed care system to join. Competition among physicians, which has traditionally been controlled through a complex set of professional norms and practices, is being replaced by competition among alternative types of organized systems. Given the reluctance of government to intervene directly, the alternatives will ultimately be shaped by forces in an only partially regulated marketplace.

Choice has been central to the development and expansion of health insurance in the United States. The first major effort in this country to apply the principles of insurance to health care costs was the plan developed by hospitals in the late 1920s and early 1930s to cover the cost of hospitalization. Hospitals were increasingly being used by the population, but people's ability to pay was rapidly deteriorating because of the widening economic depression. Hospitals created the Blue Cross insurance program not only to allow people to protect themselves from the risks of what were becoming costly hospital stays but also to ensure hospitals the revenue they needed to stay in business during the Great Depression.

Physicians soon saw the benefit to hospitals of hospital insurance, and they too developed an insurance program. It paid for in-hospital services by physicians, mostly surgery. The physician-sponsored plan, Blue Shield, and the hospital-sponsored plan, Blue Cross, eventually achieved national status and came to be known as "the Blues." Before World War II and the early postwar years, enrollment in Blue Cross/Blue Shield (BC/BS) was essentially on an individual basis. Group enrollment received its major impetus during the war years and immediately thereafter.

Because of the wage freeze during the war, employers introduced or expanded fringe benefits, which were excluded from the freeze, as a means of attracting and rewarding employees. Health insurance was one of the benefits offered. The practice of offering fringe benefits as a part of the total remuneration of employees was further expanded after the war and became a major goal of collective bargaining. It was during this period, also, that for-profit insurance companies expanded their business into the health insurance market. These companies offer what has come to be referred to as commercial health insurance plans—that is, insurance policies that are sold commercially, the same as other goods and services. By the late 1940s the dominant forms of health insurance were commercial plans and the various Blue Cross and Blue Shield plans.

By the mid-1950s, a significant proportion of higher-level employees and unionized workers were covered by health insurance, which was limited essentially to in-hospital costs and services. Commercial health insurance offered indemnity plans (i.e., plans that pay fixed dollar amounts for specifically defined services), whereas Blue Cross/Blue Shield contracted to cover a specified set of services (e.g., thirty days of hospital care in a semiprivate room, and services provided in the hospital by a physician). An employer in the private sector customarily contracted with a single carrier, either a commercial insurance company or a BC/BS organization, for a health insurance plan for its employees. For the most part, during this time period employees had no choice of plans but could choose to go to any licensed physician and any accredited hospital.

However, as employment-based health insurance expanded to include government employees, and prepaid group practice plans evolved the requirement that employers offering a PGP plan had to offer at least one other plan (commonly referred to as "dual choice"), employers increasingly came to offer a choice of plans. Choice of plans was further encouraged by Congress's passage of the Health Maintenance Organization Act in 1973. The primary objective of the act was to achieve a private sector solution to the problems of rising health care costs and inadequate access to care by stimulating the expansion of HMOs. Though that has not been achieved to the extent envisioned, the act and the legislation that followed did contribute to increased diversification in the organization and financing of medical care, as described in the previous chapter. The insurance industry and other newly created capital ventures developed a variety of competing approaches to the organization, financing, and delivery of medical care services.

Since employers usually select the plans to be offered, however, employees have to narrow their choices to those options made available by their employers. And as Klinkman (1991) noted, an employer's selection of health plans is typically made without the direct involvement of either the employees (i.e., the patients) or physicians; it may be based mainly on considerations of short-term cost/benefit to the employer and is often made without adequate or accurate information. Nonetheless, most large employers offer choices that frequently include an HMO plan when one is available in their locality, and decisions about keeping the HMO option are influenced by what employees tell their employers about their satisfaction with the plan.

We need to keep in mind, however, that the role employers play in selecting and promoting health care plans is rapidly changing. Employers are no longer passively offering multiple plans to their employees. Some are experimenting with "flexible" benefit programs that offer a "cafeteria" of benefits structured to control the employer's overall expenditures for benefits. Such programs tend to provide incentives for employees to enroll in a managed care system or assume a greater share of health care costs through higher copayments and deductibles. Some employers are experimenting with self-insurance, wherein they pay employees' medical bills directly. Self-insurance permits greater flexibility as to what health care costs the employer pays—partly because, under the health provisions of the 1974 Employee Retirement Income Security Act (ERISA), employers who self-insure are exempt from state health insurance regulations.

Still other employers are actively participating in designing health care plans and are negotiating for the lowest-priced option. Employer involvement can also be seen in a number of other ways, including the widespread use of consultants and brokers, and the establishment of vendor relationships with providers. A very recent major change in some locales is the establishment of employer purchasing cooperatives, through which large employers are seeking to become the dominant force in the market. One subtle, yet key, indicator of the changing role of employers vis-à-vis health insurance is that the function of health-plan decision making for the company, long performed by the human resources department, is now increasingly done by the financial officers. This shift changes the emphasis from managing employee benefits programs to financial management.

In the future, therefore, it is highly likely that employers and third-party payers—both private and public—will increasingly apply pressures that favor the selection of managed care options. The unrelenting rise in costs, if no other reason, will force payers to increasingly turn to managed care. It currently appears, however, that for the most part reliance will be placed on competition among alternative managed care systems, rather than on increased governmental regulation, to provide access and control costs.

Unless the financing mechanisms successfully provide for making differential payments to managed care systems on the basis of the health needs and risks of the people they enroll, the long-term viability of such systems will depend on the health status and demographic characteristics of their members. Obviously, any managed care system that hopes to survive will need to continually enroll new members to replace those who die or disenroll. But unless the financing mechanism takes the propensity to use services into account, the population of new members must not include a disproportionate number of the sickest or those most prone to use medical care services. Since the aging of even healthy members will increase the demand for health care and, as a result, drive up the costs, a "favorable" enrollment must include enough younger, healthier members to compensate for sicker persons, or persons who use health services at a higher rate than the average in the population.

The primary issue examined in this chapter is, who chooses a prepaid group practice managed care plan, and why? In figure 2.1 we present a conceptual framework for health plan choice as a way of thinking about the factors that influence the choice of a health plan and as an organizing framework for presenting our research findings and our review of the research literature on health plan choice. It has not been formally tested as a model, but it does reflect much of the conceptualization that has implicitly guided research on health plan choice, including our own studies.

The basic assumption of the model is that two major sets of factors determine or influence health plan choice. One set impacts directly on the

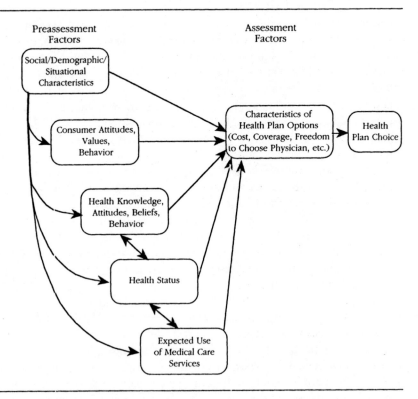

Preassessment   Assessment
Factors   Factors

Social/Demographic/
Situational
Characteristics

Consumer Attitudes,
Values,
Behavior

Characteristics of
Health Plan Options
(Cost, Coverage, Freedom
to Choose Physician, etc.)

Health
Plan Choice

Health Knowledge,
Attitudes, Beliefs,
Behavior

Health Status

Expected Use
of Medical Care
Services

Fig. 2.1. A conceptual framework for the choice of a health plan.

choice, while the effects of the other set are more indirect. The former, labeled "assessment factors" in figure 2.1, comprises characteristics of the health plan options that the chooser evaluates or assesses in the process of making a choice of plans. The other set of factors or variables comprises characteristics of the persons making the choices, or attributes of their situations, which precede the assessment process. These background characteristics are therefore labeled the "preassessment factors" in figure 2.1.

Our assumptions are that the preassessment factors directly influence or affect the assessments people make of the health plan options available to them, and that, in turn, these assessments determine health plan choice. Implicit in the model is the assumption that people have adequate knowledge or information about their various health plan options to make these assessments. In reality, of course, many people have less than adequate knowledge or may even have misconceptions about such features of the plans as what services are covered and the amount insurance will pay, and (for HMOs) how the plans operate (Mechanic, Ettel, and Davis 1990; Gallup 1991). As indicated by the arrows in the figure, the model also assumes that social, demographic, and situational factors influence or determine the assessment of health plans indirectly, through their effects on the other factors in the model. It is also assumed that health knowledge, attitudes, beliefs, and behavior, and health status, and the expected use of medical care services influence or affect one another, thus also having an indirect (and perhaps an interactive) effect or influence on health plan assessments and the choice of plan.

Our Findings

We present our findings in relation to the conceptual framework on choice and in the context of a brief review of the research literature to answer the two major questions of this chapter: Who chooses a prepaid group practice managed care plan, and why? Though our results are based on data from several sources, the primary sources are a community household interview survey conducted in 1984–85, and mail surveys of the Kaiser Permanente, Northwest Region, membership. The KPNW membership surveys have been conducted annually since 1975 by the Center for Health Research (Greenlick, Freeborn, and Pope 1988). (These are surveys of subscriber units in which the subscriber or the subscriber's spouse responds both for the unit as a whole and for individual members of the unit.) Data from the membership surveys are also used in chapter 4 when we deal with the issue of patient satisfaction with the prepaid group practice managed care plan. (See the Appendix, below, for more information about the surveys.)

Who Chooses a Prepaid Group Practice Managed Care Plan?

SOCIAL AND DEMOGRAPHIC CHARACTERISTICS

A comparison of the age and sex distribution of KPNW members with census data for the population residing in the KPNW service area is shown in figure 2.2. With some exceptions, the KPNW membership is generally similar in age and sex composition to the community population. The percentage of persons 65 years of age or older, for example, is about the same in both groups. The differences partially reflect the inclusion of the uninsured population in the census data. That is, the underrepresentation of young adults among the KPNW membership is

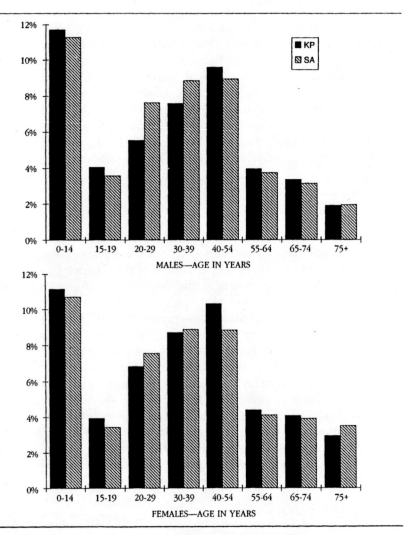

Fig. 2.2. The age and sex of the KPNW membership and of the service area *(SA)* population.
Source: Data from Kaiser Permanente Central Office 1991.

consistent with the 1984–85 community household survey that showed young, unmarried adults to be disproportionately represented among those without health insurance. Additionally, whereas the Portland metropolitan area has a lower proportion of ethnic minorities than does the total U.S. population, the representation of ethnic minorities among the KPNW membership (6.1%) is less than that in the Portland

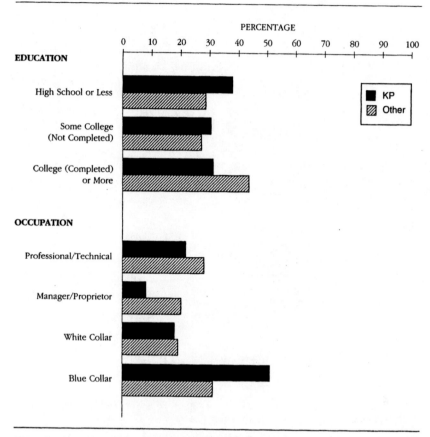

Fig. 2.3. Sociodemographic characteristics of subscribers under age sixty-five: KPNW compared with other health plans in the service area.
Source: Data from CHR 1984–85 Community Survey.

metropolitan area as a whole (8.8%). Ethnic minorities, too, are less likely to have health insurance.

In other sociodemographic characteristics KPNW subscribers are similar to subscribers to other plans. The primary differences of the subscribers under the age of sixty-five (subscribers aged sixty-five and over—virtually all covered by Medicare—have been excluded from this analysis) are to be found in the interrelated characteristics of education, occupation, income, and social class (figs. 2.3–4). By comparison with subscribers to other plans, significantly more KPNW subscribers have no more than a high school education, fewer are employed in entrepreneurial and managerial occupations, more are employed in blue-collar occupations, and fewer have a high family income. Congruent with this

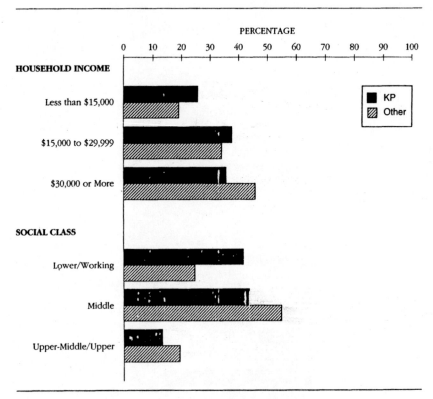

Fig. 2.4. Socioeconomic characteristics of subscribers under age sixty-five: KPNW compared with other health plans in the service area.
Source: Data from CHR 1984–85 Community Survey.

is the greater proportion of KPNW subscribers than of subscribers to other plans who report themselves as working class; subscribers to other plans more frequently report themselves as middle class and upper-middle class.

KPNW subscribers also differ from subscribers in other plans in that a greater proportion of them work for large organizations and belong to unions (fig. 2.5). Large work organizations tend to offer their employees a choice of plans that includes KPNW, and unionized workers have long had access to the KPNW plan. Among KPNW subscribers there are more who work in government and in industries related to professional and technical services, and fewer who work in retail and business services, than there are among subscribers to other plans.

Because data on demographic characteristics such as age, sex, family size, and the like are objective and relatively easily obtained, they have

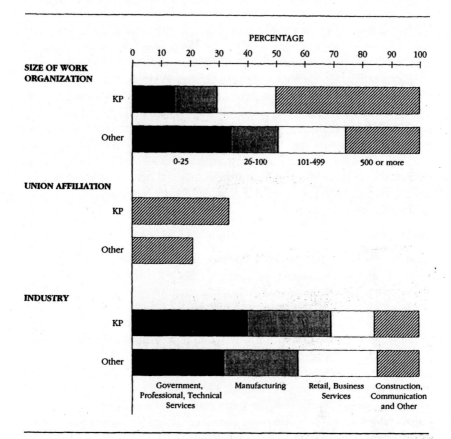

Fig. 2.5. Work-related characteristics of subscribers under age sixty-five: KPNW compared with other health plans in the service area.
Source: Data from CHR 1984–85 Community Survey.

been routinely examined in studies having to do with health plan enrollment (which now span more than twenty-five years). However, most studies comparing the social and demographic characteristics of prepaid group practice HMO plan enrollees to those of enrollees in fee-for-service plans (mostly BC/BS or the combination of BC/BS and commercial plans) have not found significant differences on most of these factors. Further, differences that have been observed in one study or a few studies have not been found by other studies. Comparisons of the studies suggest that variations in the findings are probably largely artifactual; that is, they are due to variations in the study designs, the types of populations studied (e.g., employees of a single large employer, such as a university, or members of a specific union or work group), and such things as whether the HMO is newly created, a few years old, or well established (Berki and Ashcraft 1980; Klinkman 1991).

If one takes into account the many factors affecting the findings of the various studies from the past twenty-five years and focuses on more recent data, HMO members generally appear to be highly comparable in their social and demographic characteristics to persons covered by other private health insurance. This generalization is reported by Gordon and Kaplan (1991). It is also consistent with a recent national poll (Gallup 1991), which found no significant differences in demographic characteristics between enrollees in HMO plans and those enrolled in traditional indemnity and BC/BS plans.

HEALTH STATUS

It is widely believed that HMO plans enroll healthier people than do other insurers. On the face of it, there appears to be some support for this notion. Enrolling in an HMO often requires giving up a physician with whom one has an established relationship. Sicker persons are more likely to be reluctant to do this because they are more likely to have an established relationship with a physician. Those who have never established ties to a physician, and those whose ties are involuntarily broken, do not have this constraint. Younger and healthier people are less likely to have developed strong ties to their physicians. Involuntary breaking of ties with physicians is most likely to occur when people move or change jobs—which, in turn, is also more characteristic of young people who are healthy and who use few health services.

Among the insured under the age of sixty-five, KPNW subscribers and their families do not differ significantly from enrollees in other plans with respect to their self-reported health status or their reporting of chronic or serious conditions (fig. 2.6). The majority report their family's overall health status as excellent or good. There is only a slight tendency for more KPNW subscribers to report their overall family health status as fair or poor, or mixed (i.e., some family members fair or poor, others excellent or good). In terms of their self-reports of major chronic conditions, KPNW subscribers and their families do not differ from those enrolled in the other plans. Consistent with their overall health status, most subscribers do not report chronic or serious disease for themselves or other family members. Similarity of health status is also consistent with the findings from a previously published study that found the mortality experience of KPNW members (i.e., death rates and cause of death by age and sex) to be essentially the same as that of the general Oregon population (McFarland et al. 1986).

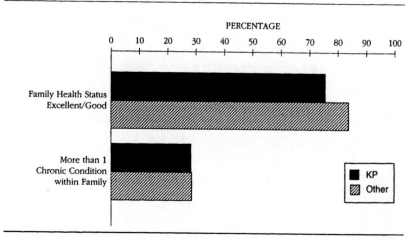

Fig. 2.6. Health status of families of subscribers under age sixty-five: KPNW compared with other health plans in the service area.
Source: Data from CHR 1984–85 Community Survey.

When asked about how they expected their membership in KPNW to affect their health, around half of the KPNW subscribers expressed the belief that their or their family's health would be better than if they were insured in some other way. From answers to open-ended questions, it appears that the major reason for believing that KPNW membership would result in better health was the belief that because of lower out-of-pocket costs (for deductibles and copayments) or broader, more comprehensive coverage, KPNW provides better access to preventive care and to care in emergencies or when one is faced with serious illness. As one survey respondent put it, "We don't have to put off going to a doctor because it costs too much. Practically everything is covered, surgery and other things."

Some studies have attempted to look at health status as a factor in health plan choice, although Bice (1975) argued that the predisposition to use services could be a better predictor of choice than health status per se. Self-reports and various utilization measures are the most commonly used measures of health status. The use of services before enrollment has also been used as a measure of the predisposition to use services (Berki and Ashcraft 1980).

Wilensky and Rossiter (1986) reviewed most of the studies on HMO enrollment from 1974 to 1986. Their focus was on the issue of self-selection and the question of whether HMOs tend to enroll healthier populations. They based their assessment primarily on self-reported health status and utilization (or claims) one year before enrollment in an

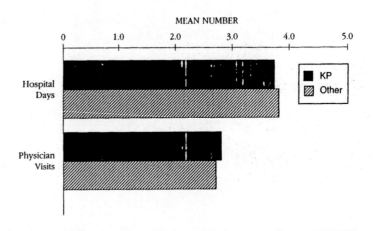

Fig. 2.7. The use of services by families of subscribers under age sixty-five: KPNW compared with other health plans in the service area.
Note: The mean numbers shown are the hospital days and physician visits per individual family member in families with hospitalizations and physician visits.
Source: Data from CHR 1984–85 Community Survey.

HMO. They concluded that earlier studies (before 1982) showed mixed results but that most of the later studies indicated that HMOs were enrolling a lower-risk (healthier) population. Luft and Miller (1988) also summarized the empirical evidence on selection bias and concluded that "HMOs are subject to some favorable selection of new enrollees according to prior health care use and cost measures, although no selection bias at all is also a common result in many studies" (Luft and Miller 1988, 110).

THE USE OR EXPECTED USE OF
MEDICAL CARE SERVICES

We found no differences between KPNW subscribers and their families and the subscribers of other plans and their families with respect to their self-reported use of medical care services (fig. 2.7). Similar proportions in the community survey reported having been admitted to a hospital during the previous twenty-four months and having visited a physician during the past year, and the number of days hospitalized and the number of office visits reported are virtually the same. These findings are the same as those reported in a recent national poll that asked enrollees in traditional and managed care plans about their use of physicians and hospitals in the previous twelve months (Gallup 1991). The utilization of services by the enrollees in the two types of plan was essentially identical.

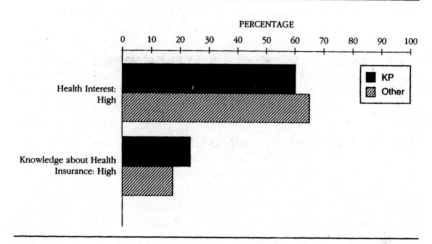

Fig. 2.8. Interest in health and knowledge about health insurance among subscribers under age sixty-five: KPNW compared with other health plans in the service area.
Source: Data from CHR 1984–85 Community Survey.

Previous studies have not been so consistent in their findings, however (Berki and Ashcraft 1980; Luft 1981; Buchanan and Cretin 1986; Klinkman 1991). Some have found that HMO enrollees tend to have had more physician visits and hospital admissions in the previous year than do enrollees in traditional plans, and other studies have shown few or no differences in prior utilization.

HEALTH ATTITUDES, KNOWLEDGE, BELIEFS, AND BEHAVIORS

KPNW subscribers were not significantly different from subscribers to other plans in terms of their expressed levels of interest in or concern with health, or in their self-reported knowledge about health insurance (fig. 2.8). There was only a slight tendency for relatively more KPNW subscribers to report being very knowledgeable about health insurance, and for a smaller proportion of KPNW subscribers than of subscribers to other plans to indicate being extremely interested in or concerned about health.

Though the difference in opinions about the role of government in health insurance is not significant, relatively more KPNW subscribers tend to favor national health insurance, and relatively fewer opt for limiting the role of government to programs for the elderly and other special-need populations, or to regulation only. It should be observed, however, that a large majority of all subscribers believe that government has a major role in health insurance.

Berki et al. (1977b) found that people with greater concern about health (identified by asking them how much they thought about their present and future health and how confident they were of continued good health) were more likely to enroll in an HMO. Metzner and Bashshur (1967) explored the relationship between beliefs about the role of government in health insurance, and choice. They observed that similarities between BC/BS and HMO enrollees were greater than differences, although a higher proportion of HMO enrollees than of BC/BS enrollees were favorably disposed toward government health insurance. Wolinsky (1976) found that heads of households who believed health care to be a right had more positive attitudes toward HMOs than did those who did not. Tessler and Mechanic (1975b) found no difference between HMO and BC/BS enrollees with respect to attitudes toward preventive services, perceived control over illness, faith in physicians, or skepticism about medical care.

CONSUMER ATTITUDES, VALUES, AND BEHAVIOR

Several approaches were taken to identify the consumer orientations of the families included in the CHR 1984–85 community survey. Questions about shopping patterns and preferences were asked to get at the trade-offs these families made between cost and quality when deciding what to buy; we determined the extent to which their shopping patterns reflected a "highbrow" rather than a mass-market orientation on the basis of their reports of which stores they most frequently patronized for personal and household goods (e.g., clothes and furniture). We defined those stores with a reputation for offering more exclusive and "upscale" products as "highbrow"; stores that offer mass-produced and "downscale" products we defined as "mass-market" stores.

Consistent with their socioeconomic characteristics, a greater proportion of KPNW subscribers than of subscribers to other plans reported that cost was a primary consideration when they shopped (fig. 2.9). The latter were more likely to report that considerations of cost versus quality depended on what was being purchased. These patterns are also reflected in the attitudes expressed toward name brands. Relatively more of the KPNW subscribers reported that products marketed under a store's own name were likely to be as good as products carrying a national brand name.

These attitudes and opinions are consonant with shopping behavior. Compared to KPNW subscribers, significantly more of those insured through other types of plans reported shopping patterns that can be

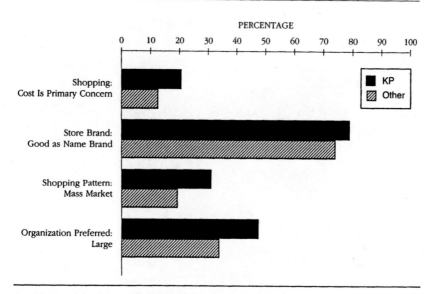

Fig. 2.9. Consumer orientations of subscribers under age sixty-five: KPNW compared with other health plans in the service area.
Source: Data from CHR 1984–85 Community Survey.

characterized as "highbrow." Relatively more KPNW subscribers reported what can be characterized as mass-market shopping patterns. These shopping patterns are consistent with the preferences expressed regarding the size of organization these families like to deal with: relatively more of the KPNW subscribers said that they preferred to patronize or deal with large organizations rather than small ones, whereas relatively more of those subscribing to other plans expressed a preference for patronizing small organizations—presumably specialty stores and enterprises offering more personalized services.

What Are the Reasons for Choosing a Prepaid Group Practice Managed Care Plan?

COST FACTORS

In the 1984–85 community survey, the major reasons given by KPNW subscribers for selecting KPNW were costs (the cost-related factors that were mentioned included more comprehensive benefits and lower out-of-pocket costs—i.e., lower copayments and/or the absence of deductibles). (See fig. 2.10.) Subscribers to other plans mentioned costs much less frequently, and more frequently reported simply that they got their

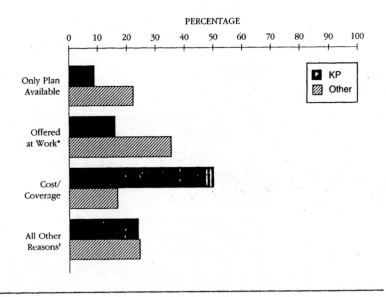

Fig. 2.10. The major reason for health plan choice by subscribers under age sixty-five: KPNW subscribers compared with subscribers of other health plans in the service area. * No further explanation given; † Choice of physician/hospital mentioned by 11.5 percent of those selecting plans other than KPNW.
Source: Data from CHR 1984–85 Community Survey.

health insurance through work (implying but not specifically indicating that it was the only plan available) or said that the health insurance they had was the only plan offered at work. These findings are highly consistent with those of a recent national poll (Gallup 1991). Nationally, managed care subscribers more frequently reported choosing their plans because of lower premiums and better coverage, whereas traditional plan subscribers more frequently reported that they chose their plan because it was the only one available. And among those who had selected their current plan within the past twelve months, managed care subscribers more frequently reported that they had done so to improve both costs and coverage.

When subscribers have been asked in the KPNW membership surveys to indicate and rate the factors that influenced their initial decision to enroll in KPNW, cost has also consistently been identified as a very important factor (fig. 2.11). The majority of KPNW subscribers have also consistently perceived KPNW benefits as more comprehensive than those of most other plans and have believed that the total costs for KPNW (i.e., premiums plus out-of-pocket costs) are less than those for

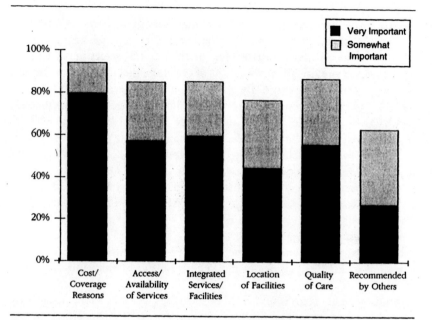

Fig. 2.11. Importance of subscribers' reasons for joining KPNW.
Source: Data from CHR Current Membership Surveys (1980, 1981, and 1982 averaged).

other plans. In the words of one survey respondent, "It [KPNW] covers all the services from surgery to allergies. Complete range of services. You get more for your money, more care. More coverage for your money."

In contrast to KPNW subscribers, subscribers to other plans cited choice of physician (and to a much lesser extent, choice of hospital) as an important reason for their selections. These findings are congruent with studies that have shown that not being able to choose their own physicians and hospitals is a major reason that people give for not selecting the HMO option (Sorensen and Wersinger 1980; Mechanic, Ettel, and Davis 1990). Persons who choose traditional plans tend to give greater importance to the freedom to choose physicians, whereas those selecting HMOs tend to give priority to cost considerations (Luft 1981; Klinkman 1991).

COVERAGE FACTORS

Because of HMOs' need to be competitive, their premiums have generally been kept in the same price range as those of the BC/BS plans in their service areas. The difference has been the greater comprehensiveness of the coverage offered by HMOs, which includes but is not limited to preventive services. In our KPNW membership surveys, comprehensiveness or range of coverage has been cited by a large proportion of subscribers as an important reason for their initial selection of KPNW. And as noted previously, the amount of coverage they receive for the cost of their premium is given by many as a major reason for selecting KPNW. One survey respondent observed that she liked the "extent of the care that is available. If they don't have it here [within KPNW] it's available elsewhere, but nevertheless through Kaiser."

Several studies, including a recent national poll (Gallup 1991), have found comprehensiveness of coverage to be cited more frequently by HMO subscribers than by subscribers in other types of plans as an important reason for selecting their plan (Moustafa, Hopkins, and Klein 1971; Davie, Goldberg, and Rowe 1974; Roghmann et al. 1975; Sorensen and Wersinger 1980; Shuttiga, Falik, and Steinwald 1984). Liberal maternity benefits have also been suggested as reasons for enrolling in HMOs (Hudes et al. 1980; Shuttiga, Falik, and Steinwald 1984).

Studies have also found HMO enrollees to use more preventive services before enrolling (indicating, perhaps, a predisposition to use preventive services) or after enrolling (Wolinsky 1976; Berki et al. 1977b; Dutton 1979), which suggests that HMO enrollees may have been attracted by the inclusion of preventive services in HMO coverage. In post-enrollment studies, however, it is difficult to say whether preventive visits are a function more of individual predisposition or of a plan's organizational characteristics (Berki et al. 1977b) or level of coverage (Luft 1981). Luft (1981) concluded, after a careful review of the existing evidence, that level of coverage—not the way in which care was organized—was the key factor. When he compared HMOs and traditional plans with similar coverage for preventive care, no differences in use could be shown. Other studies have found preventive utilization rates to be similar in HMO and in fee-for-service plans (Freeborn and Pope 1982; Gordon and Kaplan 1991).

ACCESS TO CARE

Because most people think of access to care in terms of having or not having health insurance, not much attention has been given to access as a factor in health plan choice. However, because those selecting an HMO are buying membership in a health care organization that provides or arranges for their medical care—inpatient and outpatient care, and preventive, routine, and emergency care—rather than just health insurance, they may have a different concept of access. This appears to be reflected in the reasons given for selecting KPNW. As one respondent said about KPNW, "The doctors, hospital, clinic, emergency, it's all available all the time. There's no question of availability." In our membership surveys, subscribers have indicated that KPNW's provision of physicians and facilities and the availability of medical care services through KPNW—that is, "always having a place to go for care when it is needed"—are important reasons for joining. These and other aspects of access, such as convenient locations of KPNW facilities, are mentioned by large proportions of subscribers as important reasons for joining KPNW.

Other studies have also found HMO enrollees more likely than IPA or BC/BS enrollees to give guaranteed access to services (Roghmann et al. 1975; Ashcraft et al. 1978; Sorensen and Wersinger 1980) or the availability of care at night and on weekends (Tessler and Mechanic 1975b) as reasons for joining. In one recent study, however, access was not identified as a factor affecting choice of plans (Mechanic, Ettel, and Davis 1990). The authors suggest that this is probably because most consumers assume that health insurance per se provides access to care.

THE QUALITY OF CARE

Although most Americans apparently assume that high quality is the norm for medical care in the United States, subscribers in the CHR membership surveys frequently identified quality of care as an important reason for selecting KPNW. One respondent, for example, stated: "The most important thing to me is that all the doctors concerned with Kaiser are specialists in their field." This is apparently at least part of the reason why friends, relatives, and co-workers have recommended KPNW to them. But the fact that physicians in KPNW practice as part of a group is perceived by some members as an indicator of high-quality care. To quote another respondent, "If one doctor wants the advice of another, he is there and available for expert consultation." Among those who selected a traditional plan, having a choice of physicians is also probably seen as one way of ensuring high-quality care.

Scitovsky, McCall, and Benham (1978) found IPA enrollees considerably more likely than HMO enrollees to give physician competence as a reason for joining the IPA plan, and physician incompetence as a reason for not joining the HMO plan. They also found IPA enrollees much more concerned than HMO enrollees with physician "niceness." Another study (Tessler and Mechanic 1975b) found that a very small proportion of Blue Cross enrollees gave as a reason for not joining the HMO plan its "clinic atmosphere," which probably was an expression of a judgment on quality.

OTHER PEOPLE'S INFLUENCE OR RECOMMENDATIONS

As suggested above, the importance of other people to an individual's selection of health insurance is primarily what they communicate about the attributes or consequences of the options available. That is, friends, relatives, and co-workers are sources of information, as well as repositories of opinions and attitudes, that affect an individual's behavior. The importance of others is indicated by the proportion of KPNW subscribers who cite other people's recommendations as important reasons for their selecting KPNW. Formal sources of information, such as descriptive pamphlets or other written materials, do not appear to have been major sources of information influencing the decision to select KPNW, although one respondent suggested that KPNW "should use community resources more to educate the public. They should use media advertising to advertise their services."

Metzner and Bashshur (1967) found co-workers to be the chief source of information about the HMO plan in their study and noted the importance of friends passing on information by word of mouth. Newspapers and other print media were generally felt to be the least valuable means of communication. However, Moustafa, Hopkins, and Klein (1971) found that HMO subscribers cited studying the health insurance pamphlets as their major reason for enrolling, although the advice of friends was also a major reason. One study (Mechanic, Ettel, and Davis 1990) found that people who joined an HMO were significantly more likely than those who joined a BC/BS plan to have talked about their choice with friends and co-workers who were members of the HMO.

Given our findings, we sought to determine which of the various factors was most predictive of health plan choice (fig. 2.12). By far the most important was the favorable comparison between KPNW's cost and coverage and the cost and coverage of other insurance. Additionally, being employed in a blue-collar occupation and having a mass-market shopping orientation were important in making the decision to select KPNW.

Summary and Discussion

Our findings as to who chooses a prepaid group practice managed care plan, and why, are generally very much in line with patterns reflected in the more recent research literature on health plan choice. Persons who chose KPNW are highly similar to those enrolled in traditional plans with respect to most social and demographic characteristics, as well as

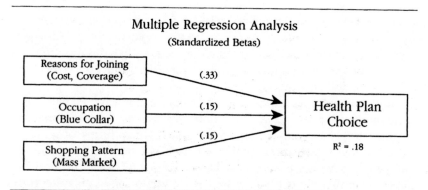

Fig. 2.12.   Significant predictors of health plan choice ($p < .01$).
Source: Data from CHR 1984–85 Community Survey.

their self-reported health status and their recent prior use of medical care services. Since KPNW has been around for more than forty-five years, and a large number of people in the community are either former or current members of KPNW (although most residents have never belonged to KPNW), it is not surprising to find this high degree of similarity.

KPNW subscribers are predominantly drawn from the middle economic stratum of society, often referred to collectively as the American middle class, and they predominantly characterize themselves as working class or middle class. Underrepresented among the KPNW membership are those highest in the social and managerial hierarchies of the community. The primary reason given for joining KPNW is cost—comprehensive coverage is provided at a cost that is the same as or lower than the price that others pay for more limited coverage. Information and recommendations from others—friends, co-workers, and relatives—are significant factors. This finding is consistent with research in the social sciences on voting and political party preference and on consumer and other behaviors, which finds that friends, relatives, and co-workers strongly influence people's preferences and choices (Katz and Lazarsfeld 1955). This body of research shows interpersonal influence and reference groups to be more important in people's decision making than information gained from newspapers, magazines, radio or television, and other mass media.

Specific, objective, and accurate information about various health plans is usually not readily available to consumers, and it is not surprising that they seek advice from friends, relatives, and others who have knowledge or experience to draw on. Mechanic (1989) reinforced this point and suggested that when information is deficient, most consumers choose on the basis of selected preference criteria conditioned by "location in the life cycle and family context, by the psychological costs of uncertainty and time required to acquire new information, and by the limits in understanding how varying plans function" (Mechanic 1989, 140).

Most communities in the United States do not have managed care plans, and most people have only vague notions regarding the differences between prepaid group practices, IPAs, and other forms of managed care. Alternatives to traditional plans have not been widely available, and people have not been exposed to or conscious of any medical care model other than the traditional fee-for-service model. In today's medical care market and environment, however, consumers are increasingly being exposed to a bewildering array of new medical care alternatives, though objective information on the performance, benefits, costs, and other attributes of these alternative ways of organizing, financing, and delivering services is still not widely available and is not disseminated in a way that enables people to make informed choices.

Advertising, which was not permissible for professional services in the past, bombards people with "sound bites" and advertisements extolling the advantages (with no mention of the disadvantages) of the various health care alternatives. The focus is on image and propaganda, and not substance or impartial facts. As Hibbard and Weeks (1989) pointed out, information for comparative shopping in health care is not readily available, and there is little evidence on how consumers would use such information in making health care decisions if it were available. Nevertheless, they recommend that both cost and quality information on various providers and health plans be made available to consumers and that increased educational efforts be made to encourage and help consumers to become better informed. These recommendations are consistent with recent recommendations of the Office of Technology Assessment calling for the development and dissemination of more objective information.

Lack of information, however, is not the primary constraint on health plan choice. Choice is constrained by various historical, social, environmental, organizational, and market forces external to the individual. These have determined the geographic distribution of managed care plans, and the number, types, and capacities of the managed care plans available in any given locale, as well as whether they are included among the options available through employment and available to Medicare and Medicaid beneficiaries.

3

Access and Continuity in Managed Care

> Everyone who is born holds dual citizenship, in the
> kingdom of the well and in the kingdom of the
> sick. Although we all prefer to use only the good
> passport, sooner or later each of us is obliged, at
> least for a spell, to identify ourselves as citizens
> of that other place.
> —Susan Sontag

Managed care is generally seen as effective in removing or lowering financial barriers to care through its comprehensiveness of coverage, limited copayments, and lack of large deductibles. Because HMOs provide physicians and facilities rather than indemnities for covered services, they also overcome the barrier of lack of medical care resources. However, many think that these barriers are replaced by organizational barriers to access and continuity of care—that is, by problems of getting into the system and by fragmented rather than continuous or coordinated care.

Some observers suggest that HMOs may make access particularly difficult for certain categories of people because the complex organizational arrangements associated with managed care may overwhelm these people and deter them from seeking necessary care. There is concern, for example, that older patients, those with serious physical and mental disabilities, and those with low income and little education may find it especially difficult to gain access to care and to obtain needed follow-up care (Lewis, Fein, and Mechanic 1976). So although financial barriers may be fewer, bureaucratic barriers that older or disadvantaged people may have greater trouble with, such as dealing with the appointment system, may limit access in HMOs (Mechanic 1976; Mechanic 1986). Some variability in access to and use of services is to be expected, but "what must particularly be guarded against is allocation of disproportionate resources to the more affluent and sophisticated patient with less medical need but higher expectations and greater persuasiveness" (Mechanic 1986, 72). According to Mechanic (1986), this is a potentially serious problem and will require ongoing attention as increasing numbers of people enroll in managed care plans.

Access to Care

Proponents of managed care argue that access to care and the distribution of services are likely to be more equitable in HMOs than in traditional fee-for-service plans, which provide narrower coverage and require higher out-of-pocket costs (Saward 1970). Under the latter plans, price and people's level of income strongly influence access and patterns of use (Hale and Hunter 1988; Jonas 1992). Proponents also assert that an HMO plan, with its comprehensive coverage and broad range of available personnel and facilities, provides access to care and produces patterns of use that are more highly related to peoples' health status or medical care needs than to their socioeconomic status.

This assertion is supported by studies that show that HMO enrollees are more likely to have a medical care contact in a given year and tend to make at least as many ambulatory visits as people enrolled in conventional fee-for-service plans (Luft 1981; Manning et al. 1984). Studies also show that HMO enrollees' access to preventive care and symptomatic care is better than or at least as good as that provided through traditional health insurance plans. Moreover, it has been found that services are distributed more equitably, with respect to both medical need and income, in HMOs than in fee-for-service arrangements (Lawrence and Jonas 1990).

These outcomes have also been observed in countries that have achieved universal coverage through national insurance (e.g., Canada) or a national health service (e.g., Great Britain). In both Canada and Great Britain, traditional inequities in access and utilization have been reversed following the introduction of universal coverage or the national health service. Before the introduction of these national programs, people lower in socioeconomic status and in poorer health were less likely to seek care and used relatively fewer health services than did those higher in socioeconomic status and in better health. Following the introduction of universal coverage, these patterns changed, and access to and the use of health care services now more closely reflect indicators of the need for care, such as health status (Muller 1986), although within these countries health status is still strongly related to socioeconomic status (Cockerham 1992).

The Continuity of Care

The HMO model is thought to reconcile the goals of equity and accessibility with cost containment, since this organizational form covers most services, including prevention, while avoiding the fee-for-service incentive to provide unnecessary services (Luft 1981; Muller 1986). HMOs have a contractual responsibility to provide or arrange for the facilities and physicians through which their members receive care. When people join an HMO, they are not just buying health insurance. They are buying access to a health care system and have a contractual right to medically necessary services.

In the group-model HMO, physicians are part of a medical group that collectively is responsible for the members of the HMO. For the most part, they work in primary care or other departments that tend to be clustered together in facilities that also usually include support services such as laboratories, x-ray services, pharmacies, and the like. Being located in close proximity, physicians can easily access one another, which helps them to coordinate care for their patients. They can readily consult with one another informally (without fear of loss of fees), as well as make formal referrals and share information through the single medical record maintained for each HMO member (which also helps eliminate duplicate tests and procedures). Since the details and the results of care by any HMO physician or provider become part of the member's medical chart, this information is available to all other clinicians who provide care to the member, including the member's primary care physician, who is formally responsible for coordinating the member's care. Because many functions are centralized, information can be exchanged between a number of contact points—the laboratory, the pharmacy, the physician's office, and the hospital. Besides contributing to efficiency and cost savings, the sharing of information, whether by means of informal consultation or by means of centralized data systems, is a vital component of coordinating care and achieving a high level of continuity of care.

Continuity of care is also the reason that most HMOs encourage members to choose a personal primary care physician—a general internist, family practitioner, or general pediatrician—and to return to that physician when care is needed. Studies have shown that having an identifiable medical provider increases people's ability to obtain medical care (Aday et al. 1993). Primary care physicians serve as gatekeepers (the physicians of first contact) and are expected to manage and integrate the process of medical care. In a model HMO, a primary care physician establishes an ongoing relationship with his or her patients, handles most of their ordinary medical problems, arranges referrals and consultations for them, admits them to the hospital, and provides follow-up care. Ideally, primary care physicians also provide basic preventive and acute care to their patients and manage the patients' chronic diseases and disabilities.

Comprehensive medical records, integrated data systems, and each patient's having a regular physician not only are basic ingredients of good care but also contribute significantly to the coordination of care and the realization of a high level of continuity of care (Donabedian 1985).

In general, fee-for-service plans (including PPOs) do not require patients to choose a primary care physician, and people can go directly to specialty services. This arrangement enhances choice of physician—and perhaps, as Rubin et al. (1993) suggested, patient satisfaction—but it can also lead to a greater use of more costly tertiary (specialty and/or subspecialty) services and is very likely to result in much discontinuity of care. In many other countries, most primary care physicians are generalists and patients must be referred to specialists by their primary care physicians. In the United States, the combination of specialty domination and fee-for-service payment leads to much extra and often unnecessary care and is one of the major reasons why U.S. costs are so high by comparison with costs in other countries. It is also the reason why continuity of care is so problematic (Relman 1992b).

A Model for Access

Andersen et al. (1983) proposed a model of access that combines characteristics of the delivery system and characteristics of individuals (see fig. 3.1). They postulated that access to the health care system "is influenced by structural characteristics of the delivery system itself and the nature of the wants, resources, and needs that potential consumers . . . bring to the care-seeking process. The realization of [access] is reflected in a population's . . . rates of utilization and in subjective descriptions of the care eventually obtained" (Andersen et al. 1983, 50).

In the model, the use of services (e.g., preventive exams, office visits, and hospital admissions) is considered an objective indicator of access. Member satisfaction with access to care, and with the care received, is considered a subjective indicator of access. Utilization and satisfaction are considered to reflect actual, or realized, access to health services. The

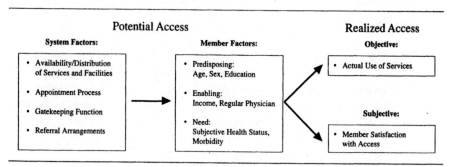

Fig. 3.1. A conceptual framework for access in managed care.
Source: Adapted from Andersen et al. 1983, 51.

availability of health care resources and the convenience aspects of access (e.g., travel time, appointment time, and waiting time in the office) are viewed as predictors of the realized outcomes (utilization and satisfaction). In this model, the ultimate proof of access is the actual use of services and resources by the people who need them—not just the availability of resources and services.

In the following section, we report our findings on access to care in KPNW. Our focus is on objective measures of access rather than on subjective aspects such as satisfaction, which we address in the next chapter. We attempt to answer the question, is access related primarily to people's need for care (as reflected by their own assessments of their health status) or to other factors, such as socioeconomic status, that traditionally affect access? That is to say, we attempt to address the concerns that have been raised regarding the capacity of managed care to provide services in an equitable way to various groups in the population.

We measure access in several ways: KPNW members' reports of appointment lag times and waiting times in the medical office; their reports of whether or not they have a regular physician; and their actual use of medical care services. In chapter 4, we will look at KPNW members' level of satisfaction with specific aspects of access as well as with overall access to care in KPNW. The membership surveys and a special research outpatient utilization data system (the Outpatient Utilization System [OPUS]) are the basic data sources for the current chapter (see Greenlick, Freeborn, and Pope 1988 and the Appendix, below, for a description of OPUS). Before we discuss our findings, however, we need to provide the reader with some additional background on the KPNW system.

How KPNW Operates

Kaiser Permanente, Northwest Region, maintains two general hospitals and seventeen medical offices (ambulatory care facilities). The medical offices are geographically dispersed throughout the area to make them accessible to the membership. Most of the medical offices provide primary care and include a pharmacy, a laboratory, and imaging (x-ray) and optical services. Some of the medical offices concentrate on specialty and subspecialty care. These tend to be centrally located but are easily accessible to most members.

KPNW's benefit structure provides comprehensive coverage for a broad range of services. The prepaid benefits have remained similar over time and currently include coverage (at a minimal out-of-pocket expense to the member) for physician, hospital, laboratory, and imaging (x-ray) services. Physical examinations, immunizations, Pap smears, mammography, and other preventive services are also covered. Drugs are provided at reduced charges and are a prepaid benefit for a significant proportion of the population, as are eyeglasses and optical services. A dental program has been integrated into some groups' coverage and now serves a population of more than 135,000 members.

In theory, each adult KPNW member is expected to choose a regular primary care physician and to return to that physician when the need for medical care arises. In practice, as we shall see later, many members do not have a regular physician (or, if they do have one, they are not aware of it) and see a variety of providers. Family practitioners and general internists provide primary care for adults, and a family can choose either a general pediatrician or a family practitioner to take care of its children. Members can choose from a large number of primary care providers (more than one hundred internists and family physicians and more than fifty pediatricians) and can change physicians if they so desire. The focal point for medical care is the physician's office, where most patients are seen by appointment (although, as discussed below, provisions are made for patients who come in without appointments).

KPNW also provides other necessary services, and these are performed by a broad range of medical specialists and other health professionals, including physician assistants, nurse practitioners, nurse-midwives, clinic, hospital, and public health nurses, social workers, laboratory and x-ray personnel, physiotherapists, pharmacists, optometrists, and mental health professionals. A range of educational, screening, diagnostic, treatment, and rehabilitation services are available. The medical care program also provides preventive care and long-term follow-up.

Every KPNW member has a single, comprehensive medical record, and every contact an individual makes with the medical care system is recorded on this unit chart. Whenever a patient has a scheduled appointment at an ambulatory care facility (medical office), his or her record is delivered to the attending physician to be available at the time of the appointment.

Members do not have direct telephone access to their physicians in this medical care system. Rather, a member must call and leave a message, and the call will be returned by the physician or the physician's nurse. In most facilities, an advice nurse is available who can speak with the patient over the phone and, if necessary, arrange for the patient to come in and be seen by his or her physician or another appropriate provider.

KPNW, like most HMOs, has a computerized appointment system, and members are expected to make regularly scheduled appointments for non-emergency conditions or routine care. The intent of the system is to make the management of a large medical practice easier and more efficient. Appointments can be made by phone or in person at each ambulatory care facility. Preventive care is also arranged by appointment and can be provided by the patient's physician or by special health appraisal units. A patient with an acute problem can be seen without an appointment and will be seen by his or her own physician if the physician is available and has an open slot. If not, arrangements can be made for the patient to see another available physician in the same unit, or the patient can be referred to a special unit for urgent care. Emergency care is available at all hours at either of the two KPNW hospitals.

Our Findings

Access: Appointment Lag and Waiting Time in the Facility

Most of those responding to the 1989 membership survey reported that the usual waiting time for routine appointments was two weeks or less and that on average they had to wait less than fifteen minutes in the medical office (figs. 3.2–3). When we analyzed the data by age, gender, socioeconomic status, and perceived health status, no major differences in waiting time were found. Access—as measured by appointment lag and waiting time in the office—did not vary greatly by any of these characteristics. The assumption that certain groups, such as older people or people with low incomes, have special problems in obtaining access does not seem to be supported by these data.

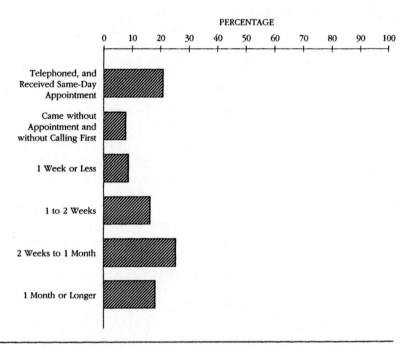

Fig. 3.2. The scheduling of members' most recent office visit to KPNW.
Source: Data from CHR 1989 Current Membership Survey.

However, the overall process for obtaining care is fairly complex and can take considerable time for most members (fig. 3.4). The average time (self-reported in the 1991 survey of office visits) consumed by telephoning to determine if a visit was needed and making an appointment was seventeen minutes. At the time of the visit, the check-in procedure, waiting time, and nurse services (checking weight, blood pressure, etc.) took on average about twenty-six minutes in all. The visit with the physician usually took around fifteen to sixteen minutes. Once the physician visit was over, patients often had to perform some additional activities such as scheduling follow-up appointments and getting support services (e.g., prescriptions, lab tests, or x rays). Thus, the entire visit-related process can take well over an hour.

Some empirical studies comparing actual appointment lags and waiting times in the office have generally found that HMO members, once they have an appointment, wait less in the office and are more satisfied with this aspect of access than patients in fee-for-service plans. However, HMO members have to wait longer to obtain appointments, whether for primary or specialty care (Luft 1981; Williams and Torrens

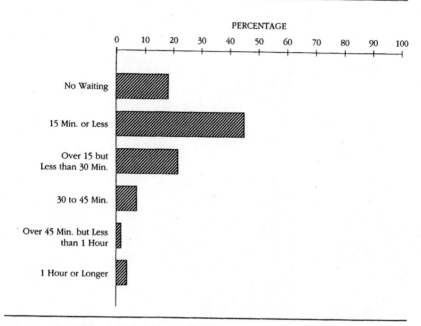

Fig. 3.3. Members' waiting time in KPNW medical office at most recent visit. *Source:* Data from CHR 1989 Current Membership Survey.

1993). These differences reflect differences between the scheduling practices in HMOs and those in fee-for-service practices. HMOs have to meet the needs of a defined population and must try to keep their physicians fully occupied by maintaining full-time appointment schedules.

In fee-for-service practice, many physicians try to squeeze in most acute and urgent cases during the course of the work day. This leads to overbooking and longer patient waiting times in the office, but it minimizes appointment lags. Physicians are likely to have to work longer hours to take care of the additional patients—a major source of dissatisfaction for many fee-for-service physicians—but this overbooking helps the physicians to achieve their income goals (Mechanic 1975; Luft 1981). These findings are by no means universal, however, since some studies have found no significant differences between prepaid plans (HMOs) and fee-for-service plans with respect to either appointment waits or waiting time in the office (Held and Reinhardt 1980).

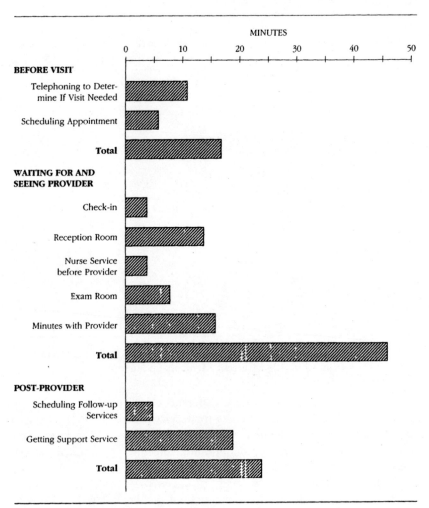

Fig. 3.4. KPNW members' visit-related process time for most recent office visit. *Source:* Data from CHR 1991 Medical Office Visit Survey.

Access: What Use Do Subscribers Make of KPNW?

The percentage of persons who receive health services in a given time period is often used as a proxy measure of access to care. In this section we compare the characteristics of those KPNW subscribers who made at least one ambulatory contact (office visit) in a twenty-four-month period with the characteristics of those who did not make a contact. Another commonly used measure of access is the volume of visits (number of office visits per person per year). We also analyze factors that affect the number of ambulatory care visits made by KPNW subscribers.

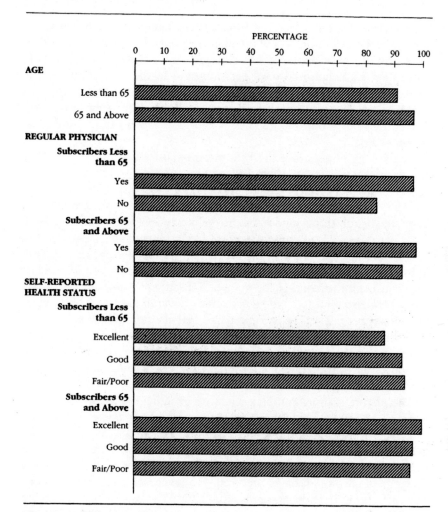

Fig. 3.5. KPNW subscribers making at least one office visit in the past twenty-four months.
Source: Data from CHR 1985 Current Membership Survey and Outpatient Utilization Study (OPUS).

Overall, it appears from our survey data that more than 90 percent of KPNW subscribers under sixty-five years of age, and 97 percent of those sixty-five years of age and older, made at least one contact with the medical care system during 1985–86 (fig. 3.5). KPNW subscribers averaged about five office visits per year. For the United States as a whole in the same time period, 85 percent of the population (all ages) saw a physician at least once, and the average person made 5.3 office visits

(USDHHS 1988; Lawrence and Jonas 1990). The striking difference is in the use of the hospital: KPNW members averaged less than four hundred short-stay hospital days per one thousand individuals, compared with more than eight hundred days per thousand in the U.S. population in 1986 (USDHHS 1988; Kaiser Permanente 1990; Lawrence and Jonas 1990). Since 1986, hospital utilization has been decreasing in the U.S. population, but group-model HMOs still have lower rates than do fee-for-service plans.

In the U.S. population, the rate of ambulatory care usage varies by age, gender, race, income, insurance coverage, and whether one has a regular source of care (Lawrence and Jonas 1990; NCHS 1992; Aday et al. 1993). In KPNW, the demographic factors of age, gender, and perceived health status tend to be the main predictors of use (figs. 3.5–7). That is to say, older people are more likely than younger people, and females are more likely than males, to contact the medical care system. Subscribers in fair or poor health are more likely than those in good or excellent health to contact the system. Subscribers who tend to contact the system also tend to have higher rates of overall use (total office visits per person per year). The income and social class of KPNW subscribers is generally unrelated to their making contact with the medical care system or to their rates of overall use of services. Education, however, does affect utilization in that subscribers with more education tend to use more services (fig. 3.7).

The picture is more complex when we examine the use of preventive services or services within specific disease categories, but age, gender, and perceived health status still tend to be important predictors of access to and use of services (figs. 3.8–10). As might be anticipated, perceived health status and the use of services are most strongly related within the category of chronic diseases (fig. 3.9). However, perceived health status also affects utilization patterns for KPNW subscribers with acute conditions—those with fair or poor health are more likely to contact the medical care system and tend to use more services on the average (fig. 3.8).

Income and perceived social class are not important determinants of access in any of the disease categories. Educational level, however, does affect subscribers' use both of preventive services and of services for acute conditions (figs. 3.8 and 3.10). Subscribers with more education are more likely to make a contact than are those with less education, and use more preventive and acute care services. Perceived health status is not related to the use of preventive services.

KPNW subscribers with a regular physician are more likely to contact the medical care system and have higher rates of use (figs. 3.5–6). We

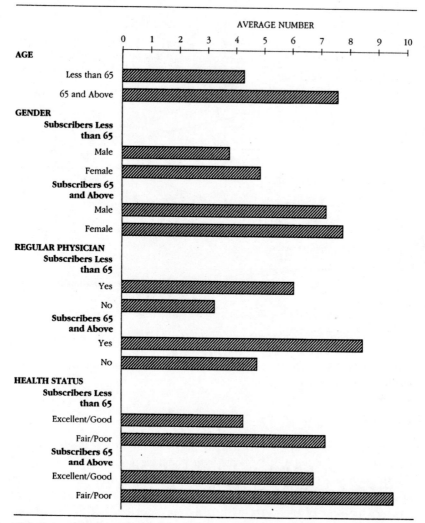

Fig. 3.6. KPNW subscribers' average number of office visits during past twenty-four months.
Source: Data from CHR 1985 Current Membership Survey and Outpatient Utilization Study (OPUS).

cannot infer from our cross-sectional data that having a regular physician causes better access. Older subscribers and/or those with poorer health use the system to a greater extent and therefore tend to establish regular ties with a specific provider. Thus, these subscribers' higher utilization rates may reflect their health status—not the fact that they have a regular physician. Other studies, however, have shown that

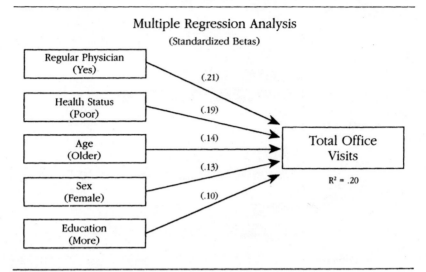

Fig. 3.7. Significant predictors of KPNW subscribers' access to ambulatory care ($p < .05$).
Source: Data from CHR 1985 Current Membership Survey and Outpatient Utilization Study (OPUS).

having a regular provider directly influences the decision to seek care (Kuder and Levitz 1985).

Continuity of Care: Who Has a Regular Physician?

In the membership surveys, we asked, "Do you and others in your family covered by KP have a KP doctor you consider your regular doctor?" More than 50 percent of subscribers and more than 60 percent of spouses of subscribers reported having a regular physician; and more than 75 percent of members with children reported that their children had a regular physician. In general, those KPNW subscribers with a regular physician tend to have poorer health—those who report fair or poor health are more likely than those reporting excellent or good health to have a regular physician (fig. 3.11). Age and frequent use of the health care system are also associated with having a regular physician. The majority of members report having a regular physician if they are over age forty or if they have had six or more visits in the past year (a proxy for poorer health status). Those with lower income and less education are also more likely to report that they have a regular physician (fig. 3.11). But these groups also tend to have poorer health than do subscribers who have higher income and more education (fig. 3.12). In

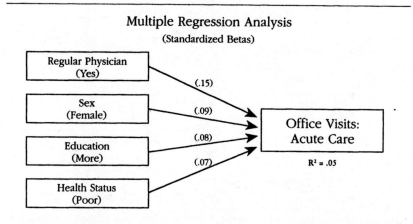

Fig. 3.8. Significant predictors of KPNW subscribers' access to acute care ($p < .05$).
Source: Data from CHR 1985 Current Membership Survey and Outpatient Utilization Study (OPUS).

general, then, those with greater need (poorer health status) tend to have a regular physician in this managed care plan.

In the general research literature, some studies suggest that when access is measured by asking people whether they have a regular provider, HMO-type managed care plans provide less access than do fee-for-service plans (Luft 1981; Williams and Torrens 1993). That is,

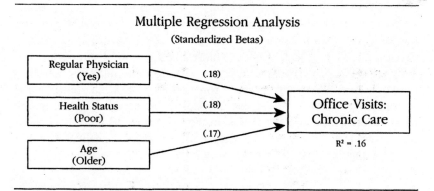

Fig. 3.9. Significant predictors of KPNW subscribers' access to chronic disease care ($p < .05$).
Source: Data from CHR 1985 Current Membership Survey and Outpatient Utilization Study (OPUS).

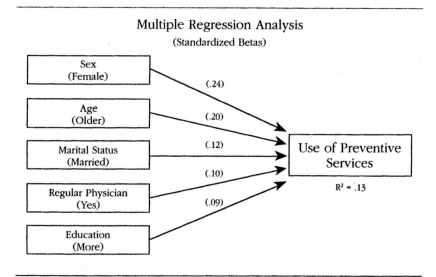

Fig. 3.10. Significant predictors of KPNW subscribers' access to preventive care ($p < .05$).
Source: Data from CHR 1985 Current Membership Survey and Outpatient Utilization Study (OPUS).

compared with patients in fee-for-service plans, HMO members are less likely to report that they have a regular physician or a personal physician. However, many HMO members consider their managed care system to be their regular source of care and, when seeking care, tend to use whatever physician or provider is available.

A lack of a regular physician tends to reflect a person's health status and/or his or her short time with the plan: persons in excellent health less frequently report having a regular physician. As members age and/or develop health problems, they are more likely to establish ongoing ties with particular primary care physicians. Younger and healthier members (and new members) may not need to—and may not even feel that it is desirable to—choose a regular physician or establish an ongoing relationship with a specific physician. For example, 20 percent of those who report that they do not have a regular physician in KPNW say that having a regular physician is not very important.

Summary and Discussion

Access to care in the KPNW managed care system is primarily a function of age, gender, and perceived health status (i.e., the need for care).

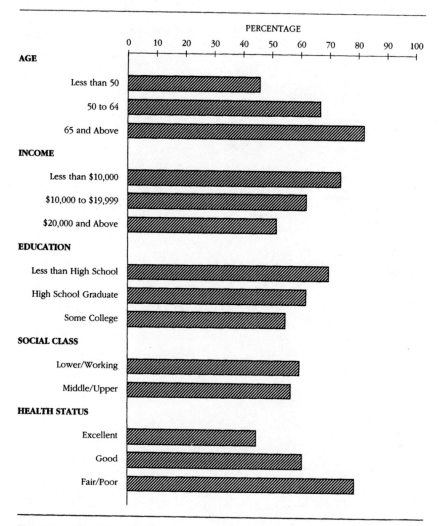

Fig. 3.11. KPNW subscribers reporting that they have a regular physician. *Source:* Data from CHR 1985 Current Membership Survey.

Socioeconomic status (income and/or social class) is not related to appointment lag times, office waiting times, whether people contact the medical care system, or the number of services received. In this sense, KPNW seems to be a fairly equitable system.

An exception is preventive care—members with more education use more preventive services—even in this system where financial and other barriers are removed. This finding is consistent with many other studies and holds across all types of health plans. Although HMOs tend to do

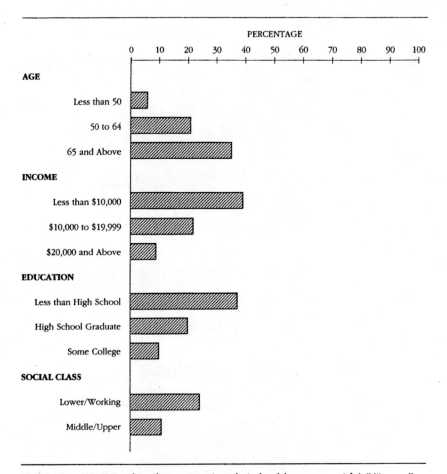

Fig. 3.12. KPNW subscribers reporting their health status as "fair"/"poor." *Source:* Data from CHR 1985 Current Membership Survey.

better than fee-for-service programs in achieving recommended levels of preventive care, they have the potential to achieve much more in the area of disease prevention and health promotion. HMOs need to develop more effective population-based preventive strategies and programs aimed at high-risk groups if equity is to be achieved in the area of prevention. Further, if health maintenance organizations are really going to live up to their name they will need to improve the overall health status of the various groups they serve, particularly those with less education and income.

Richard Weinerman, a respected clinician and an early advocate of prepaid group practice, observed that this form of delivery had achieved many organizational advantages for physicians but that clinical medicine was still largely oriented to individual practice. His observations seem as relevant today as they did a quarter of a century ago:

> Perhaps most disappointing has been the hesitation on the part of most medical groups to effect changes in the "way of life" of the medical team itself. This would involve acceptance by the group as a whole of collective responsibility for the health of its patients or members. This means actively reaching out into the community of the apparently healthy for screening and early detection. It means identification and special protection for those at specific risk of disease. It implies particular concern for those patients who do not use the service, and for those who break appointments or fail to comply with prescribed regimens. It infers as much concern with rapport as with diagnostic labels, as much concern with education as prescription. (Weinerman 1969, 30)

4

Patient Satisfaction with
Managed Care

> Don't ask the doctor; ask the patient.
> —Yiddish Proverb

The patient's viewpoint is only one element in the appraisal of managed care as a social enterprise, but it is an important one, since managed care will ultimately be judged by whether it satisfies those it serves. Until recently, however, the patient's perspective has largely been ignored in medical care planning and evaluation (Aharony and Strasser 1993). In this chapter we focus on how patients evaluate their experiences with this prepaid group practice managed care system and on their level of satisfaction with various aspects of care in this setting.

Studies of satisfaction/dissatisfaction with medical care in the general American population show that most people are satisfied with their medical care and their type of health plan but that an ever increasing proportion are dissatisfied with the cost of care (Hall and Dornan 1988a; Hall and Dornan 1988b; Blendon 1989; Hall and Dornan 1990; Gallup 1991). People are generally more satisfied with the technical aspect of medical treatment than with accessibility and the interpersonal component of care. Most complaints have to do with cost, accessibility, and the impersonality of the service or of the provider—not with the technical quality. Of course, among the uninsured cost and access are the major sources of dissatisfaction. As early as the late 1970s, a nationwide survey showed three-fourths of the respondents agreeing that there is a crisis in health care in the United States (Robert Wood Johnson Foundation 1978). Yet only 10 percent expressed dissatisfaction with the quality of care, whereas around 40 percent indicated dissatisfaction with costs and accessibility.

Though more recent surveys have found a greater proportion of Americans expressing dissatisfaction with both cost and access to care, satisfaction with technical quality remains high (Blendon 1989). Lay people feel competent to make judgments about costs, accessibility, convenience, and the like, but they feel less competent to make judgments about professional knowledge and technical competence. Most appear to assume that physicians have the requisite technical knowledge and competence. This is congruent with the content of medical education, which emphasizes technical competence and gives little attention to those elements that have to do with practice settings, patients' psychosocial needs, and the development of the interpersonal skills requisite to good physician-patient relationships.

A number of analysts suggest that the growth of managed care plans may lead to growing dissatisfaction among patients. There are several reasons for this assumption. Managed care is still new and unfamiliar to most Americans. Solo fee-for-service medical practice is perceived as the basic model of care, and people's perceptions shape their expectations (even though the model represents an idealized view of fee-for-service practice and of the family physician). The concepts of the "family doctor" and of each individual's right to choose a personal physician are firmly embedded in the American psyche even though many Americans lack such choice and have never had a regular physician.

In managed care, patients have less choice of physicians and less influence over physicians. Physicians who practice in HMOs tend to be oriented to their colleagues and to the organization, which provides their income, equipment, staff, and other resources. Compared with fee-for-service settings, managed care settings allow patients less influence, and physicians may resist patient requests that are not congruent with professional standards and criteria. This situation may result in a better quality of care from a technical perspective, but it can also lead to patient dissatisfaction (Freidson 1960; Luft 1981). Patients may feel that their needs and preferences have been ignored. Further, patients' preconditioned attitudes about "socialized medicine," the "charity clinic," and the "captive" patient may be carried over and may adversely affect their views when they become members of managed care plans, particularly large staff- or group-model HMOs (Weinerman 1964). In fact, one challenge to managed care is the need to satisfy a diverse and heterogeneous population. The image that some have is that HMOs are good for the working class or the mass of the middle class but that they won't work for either low-income racial/ethnic minorities or the upper-middle-income group of professionals and business executives.

In contrast to fee-for-service practice, which patients feel is more accommodating to their wants, HMOs may be perceived by patients as forcing them to conform to the organization's rules and procedures. These perceptions may not be supported by objective data but can nonetheless lead to patterns of behavior that reinforce these beliefs. The concept of the self-fulfilling prophecy is well known in social science and is an important determinant of human behavior (Merton 1968).

In fee-for-service practice, physicians depend on attracting enough patients to maintain a viable practice. Under these circumstances, physicians are less subject to influence by colleagues but more responsive to patients' wishes (even though the patients' requests may not always make sense or be justifiable from a purely technical perspective). Thus, the quality of care may suffer but patients are happier (Freidson 1960; Donabedian 1969; Luft 1981). Because of these differences between organized systems and fee-for-service practice, managed care may result in more dissatisfaction among patients, especially among those higher in socioeconomic status, who expect more deferential treatment from others (Luft 1981; Mechanic 1986). As the physician Richard Weinerman stated it: "The physician [in managed care] accepts the role of analytic and detached scientist—particularly when reinforced by the colleague-oriented professionalism of the medical group. The patient, on the other hand—alienated in an impersonal society, threatened by his illness, confused by the health center complex—seeks personal involvement and reassurance from 'his' doctor" (Weinerman 1967, 164).

To what extent are these assumptions supported by research? The majority of studies comparing the satisfaction of enrollees in HMO plans with that of people who join more traditional plans have compared enrollees in group-model HMOs with enrollees in traditional indemnity plans or Blue Cross/Blue Shield. These studies generally show that most people are satisfied with their health plan, regardless of type of plan. When asked about specific features of care, however, HMO enrollees are more likely than enrollees in traditional plans to complain about, or to be less satisfied with, waiting times for appointments, inability to see one's own physician, inadequate explanations by physicians, lack of interest in the patient as a person, and problems with physician-patient relationships generally (see, e.g., Rubin et al. 1993). These views are balanced by strong expressions of respect for the technical quality of care and by very high levels of satisfaction with coverage and out-of-pocket costs (Weinerman 1967; Donabedian 1969; Luft 1981; Murray 1987; Murray 1988).

Whereas the implicit assumption of the studies is that plan characteristics are the reasons for variations in patient satisfaction, differences in the characteristics of the people selecting the alternative plans—not features of the plans themselves—could account for the variations. That this is probably not the case is demonstrated by a more recent study (Davies et al. 1986) that randomly assigned subjects to fee-for-service practice and to managed care (a staff-model HMO). The findings are basically congruent with those of the other studies reported above. The typical person assigned to the HMO was less satisfied overall than were the persons assigned to fee-for-service. The length of appointment waits, the availability of the hospital, and the continuity of care favored fee-for-service, but coverage, costs, and waiting time in the medical office favored the HMO.

More recent data challenge some of the findings from the earlier studies. For example, a recent national poll (Gallup 1991) found enrollees in traditional BC/BS and indemnity plans and enrollees in managed care plans to be equally satisfied overall with their respective plans. And of the twelve specific dimensions examined (having to do with quality, access, convenience, etc.), enrollees in the two types of plans were equally satisfied on ten; on the other two (the amount patients had to pay for physician office visits, and the inconvenience of or the time required for paperwork), enrollees in managed care plans were significantly more satisfied. For both types of plan, enrollees were least satisfied with how their respective plans dealt with their problems and complaints. Another recent national study reported that a larger proportion of enrollees in managed care plans than of those enrolled in BC/BS and commercial plans expressed satisfaction with their health plans (Jensen 1992).

As might be expected, then, studies of individual HMOs show members making positive evaluations of costs and financial coverage and expressing high levels of satisfaction with the technical quality of care (Pope 1978; Luft 1981; Rosko and Broyles 1988). And not surprisingly, overall satisfaction is strongly related to convenience and to access to care. Whether or not a member has a personal physician, the likelihood of being able to see one's own physician, and the wait for an appointment significantly affect overall satisfaction. Other important predictors of overall satisfaction include members' satisfaction with the knowledge, ability, interest, and attention of the HMO physicians. In terms of membership characteristics, studies of both HMO plans and traditional plans consistently find age predictive of satisfaction; older members are more satisfied than are younger members (Weinerman 1964; Pope 1978; Luft 1981; Gallup 1991; Aharony and Strasser 1993).

A framework for conceptualizing the factors that influence or determine patient satisfaction with HMOs is presented in figure 4.1. Four major factors or sets of factors are assumed to have a major influence on patient satisfaction. These include the patients' social and demographic characteristics; their knowledge about health and their health-related attitudes, beliefs, and behavior; their health status; and their use of medical care services. Each of these sets of factors is conceptualized as

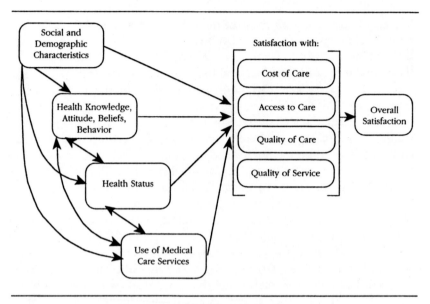

Fig. 4.1. Conceptual framework for patient satisfaction with cost, access, and the quality of care and service in a managed care system.

having a direct influence on patient satisfaction. Most are conceptualized as also having an indirect effect through their influence on other factors or variables, as indicated by the arrows in figure 4.1.

As was the case with the model presented in chapter 2, neither our own research on health plan choice and patient satisfaction nor that of others has been explicitly model-based and designed to test formal hypotheses. But models such as this have been implied in the research on these topics. We offer the models only as frameworks for helping to understand the issues we are attempting to address regarding managed care.

Our Findings

We have studied member satisfaction in Kaiser Permanente, Northwest Region, for more than twenty years. Subsequent to an extensive personal interview survey conducted in 1970–71 (which attained a 92% response rate) and the piloting, or testing, in 1974, of a mail survey for studying membership satisfaction, mail surveys of random samples of KPNW subscribers—the Current Membership Survey series—have been conducted annually since 1975. A second series of annual mail questionnaire surveys—the Surveys of Medical Office Visits—was instituted in 1991 to supplement the Current Membership Surveys. For the medical office visit surveys, a random sample of visits to each medical facility is selected weekly for a postvisit mail survey of those making the visit (or, for younger children, the parents).

The purpose of the visit survey is to obtain patients' evaluations of their visits to physicians and other providers soon after the visits. Though both surveys focus on patient satisfaction, the visit survey asks about the appointment lag associated with the specific visit, and about the quality of the care and service provided during the visit. The membership survey asks subscribers to generalize about their experience with KPNW in terms of their satisfaction or dissatisfaction with various aspects of access to care, quality of care and service, cost of care, and coverage. In the membership survey, subscribers have also been asked about the problems they and their family members have encountered in their use of KPNW, and about the use they and their family members have made of services outside KPNW (see the Appendix, below, for more details on the surveys).

Access to care and the quality of care and service are primarily attributes of KPNW as a medical care delivery system, whereas costs and coverage of health care services are primarily attributes of KPNW as an insurance system. Though these are closely intertwined, and define a managed care system, from the perspective of members they are potentially independent sources of satisfaction or dissatisfaction.

Though there is some variation from year to year in the findings from the membership surveys, the patterns of satisfaction and dissatisfaction with KPNW regarding cost of care, access to care, and quality of care and service have been highly consistent across time. Below, we describe these patterns for the subscriber population as a whole. This is followed by a discussion of patient satisfaction with specific visits. Then we examine the relationship between overall satisfaction and various characteristics of the patients, as suggested by the model in figure 4.1, to identify those social, demographic, and other characteristics of subscribers that best explain variations in satisfaction. The final section deals with behavioral indicators of dissatisfaction—the use of services outside the plan, and disenrollment.

The Cost of Care

We first look at satisfaction with the cost of care because, as we observed in chapter 2, cost is a major reason for people's choosing KPNW rather than other insurance options. In our membership surveys, we have

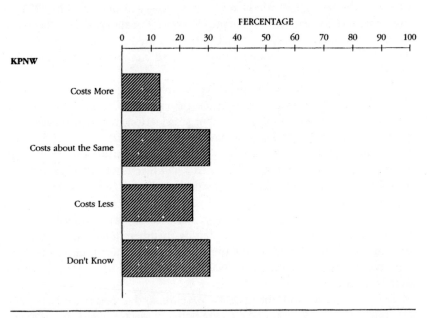

FERCENTAGE

Fig. 4.2. KPNW subscribers' comparison of the costs of the premium for KPNW with the premium costs of other health insurance plans.
Source: Data from CHR 1992 Current Membership Survey.

routinely asked subscribers to rate their satisfaction with the cost of premiums and with out-of-pocket expenses (copayments) as well as their satisfaction with total costs relative to benefits. As one of our survey respondents succinctly put it, "I like the cost most of all."

Subscribers have also been asked how they think costs for KPNW members compare with costs for people covered by other types of insurance. With regard to premiums, a large minority report not knowing how KPNW compares, reflecting the fact that most are enrolled through their employers, who pay part or all of their health insurance premiums (fig. 4.2). Of those who express an opinion, only a small minority report KPNW to be more costly. Most report the KPNW premium as being the same as that of other plans, or less costly. In terms of out-of-pocket costs, a large minority consistently report that KPNW is less costly. The majority also have consistently reported that when premiums and out-of-pocket costs are combined, KPNW members pay less for medical care services than do others (fig. 4.3). One survey respondent summed up his position this way: "I like the idea of not having to pay a huge amount for something major. . . . I was in the

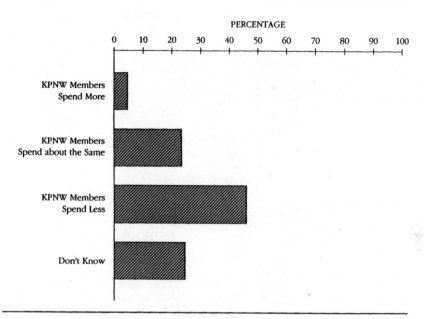

PERCENTAGE

Fig. 4.3. KPNW subscribers' comparison of total medical care costs with those for members of other health insurance plans.
Source: Data from CHR 1992 Current Membership Survey.

hospital with appendix for 21 days and almost all my expenses were taken care of by my premiums."

When asked specifically about their level of satisfaction with the total costs of care (premiums plus out-of-pocket costs), a very large majority report being "satisfied" or "very satisfied," and only a very few report being "very dissatisfied" (fig. 4.4). Because cost is a primary reason for selecting KPNW, one might assume that lower-income subscribers would be more satisfied with overall cost. But this is not the case. Higher-income subscribers and those subscribers and their families making more visits are more satisfied with the overall cost of care in KPNW.

Access to Care

Several dimensions of access have been routinely investigated in the KPNW membership surveys. These include the appointment-making process, getting appointments within the desired time period, contacting physicians by telephone, getting care without an appointment and on nights and weekends, getting care in an emergency, and getting preventive care.

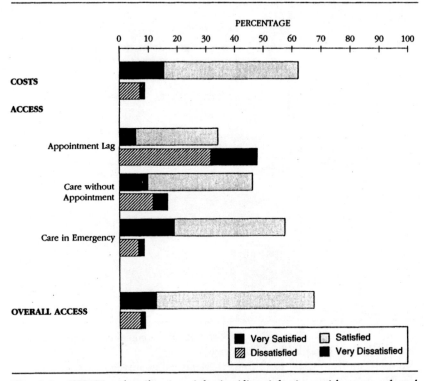

Fig. 4.4. KPNW subscribers' satisfaction/dissatisfaction with costs of and access to care.

Note: Not shown is the percentage of respondents who selected the "neutral" response on the rating scale to indicate that they had no opinion on the item being rated. These tended to be newer or young KPNW subscribers and others with limited experience in using KPNW.

Source: Data from CHR 1992 Current Membership Survey.

Dissatisfaction with access is greatest for the telephone appointment-making process, for the appointment lag time (the time between scheduling the appointment and the date of the appointment), and for non-emergency care without an appointment. One respondent expressed his frustration by saying, "One thing I don't care for is—like when you call in, they want to know if you're sick, or if you think you're sick, or if you're real bad off. When I call I usually have a reason." There is much less dissatisfaction with access to care at nights or on weekends, in emergencies, or for preventive services. Members are consistently less satisfied with the amount of time spent on the phone getting through to the appointment clerks and with the appointment lag time than with other aspects of access.

Given the relatively high levels of dissatisfaction with some aspects of access, one might expect dissatisfaction with overall access to be equally high. But this is not the case. A possible explanation emerges from responses to open-ended questions asking subscribers what they especially "like" and "dislike" about KPNW. Prominent dislikes are the waiting times on the telephone when making appointments and the appointment lag time, but these are often qualified by subscribers' descriptions of what they like: for instance, "In a real emergency or when you really need medical care, there is always a place you can go anytime of the day or night." Or a subscriber may say that access to care for routine needs is often difficult but that "if you're really sick, you'll get taken care of in KP."

Satisfaction with overall access is higher among those making more visits to KPNW, among older subscribers, among lower-income subscribers, and among healthier subscribers.

The Quality of Care and Service

Two dimensions of quality are of great importance to patients. One has to do with physicians' medical knowledge and technical skills and the other with physicians' communication and interpersonal skills (Donabedian 1985). In the membership surveys, KPNW subscribers have been asked about their satisfaction with each of these aspects of care.

A large majority have consistently expressed satisfaction with the technical knowledge, ability, and competence of the physicians in KPNW (fig. 4.5). In the words of one survey respondent: "I think they [KPNW] have a fabulous medical staff . . . they know what they're doing. They are specialists in their field." Or, as another respondent put it, "You don't have to worry about being seen by interns or residents or doctors that are in training. You're seen by a specialist. A full-fledged doctor. You're not practiced upon by residents or interns or that sort of thing."

Most members are also satisfied with the personal interest and attention they receive from KPNW physicians, with the amount of time the physicians spend with them, and with the amount of explanation or information provided by the physicians. One older respondent expressed her view by saying, "They [the doctors] are just great with me. . . . They don't seem impersonal. It seems as though I'm the patient for the moment. They don't seem distracted. I feel real at ease." A middle-age woman reported, "As a rule most of the doctors down there [at KPNW] are very conscientious with you. They take a lot of pains with you." And a younger middle-aged man said, "I like the doctors I've been in association with. They take an interest in you personally. You get more

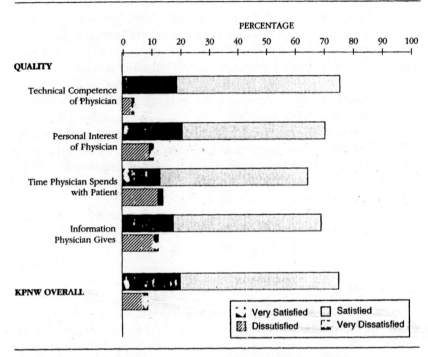

Fig. 4.5. KPNW subscribers' satisfaction/dissatisfaction with the quality of care and with KPNW overall.
Note: Not shown is the percentage of respondents who selected the "neutral" response on the rating scale to indicate that they had no opinion on the item being rated. These tended to be newer or young KPNW subscribers and others with limited experience in using KPNW.
Source: Data from CHR 1992 Current Membership Survey.

than just a prescription." The findings are similar with respect to satisfaction with the services and behavior of nurses and other medical office support personnel: "The doctors are friendly, the nurses are friendly. Everyone concerned is friendly," according to one survey respondent.

Satisfaction with the quality of care is greater for subscribers higher in self-reported social class, for persons making more visits, and for those in better health. Satisfaction with the interpersonal dimensions of the services is higher for older people and for those making more visits to KPNW.

Likes and Dislikes

As noted above, KPNW subscribers have also been asked what they particularly like and dislike about KPNW. Their "likes" included not only the cost-related factors discussed above and the lack of paperwork (e.g., insurance papers and claims forms) in KPNW but also a pattern that might be labeled "the mall phenomenon": a broad range of services (e.g., primary and specialty care) and facilities (e.g., a pharmacy, a laboratory, and an optical shop) in one convenient location with on-site parking. One respondent noted, "I like the pharmacy and the fact that everything is in one spot. The lab, x-rays, anything you need. . . . It doesn't mean repeated appointments or having to travel from place to place."

Not surprisingly, the pattern of "dislikes" had mostly to do with access. A forty-year-old woman respondent claimed, "It's getting so crowded now, to get an appointment you have to nearly be dead to get in to see somebody." Another respondent, a young man, said, "Half the time by the time you can get a doc . . . it's cleared up, and in an emergency situation you can't see your own doctor." The major dislikes were the time spent on the telephone making appointments and the lag time between the initial call to schedule an office visit for routine care, and the resulting appointment date. Negative comments about the quality of the service or care received were much less frequent.

Satisfaction with Recent Visits

In comparison to members' ratings of satisfaction or dissatisfaction with access and quality of care generally, members are much more satisfied when reporting on specific visits. The majority of members reporting on specific visits believed that the appointment lag was appropriate (fig. 4.6). A very large majority were also satisfied or very satisfied with the physician's or provider's "technical competence, skill, and ability," with the "amount of time the provider spent" with them during the visit, with the "amount of personal interest shown by the provider," and with the visit overall (fig. 4.7). When asked to evaluate the overall quality of "the care and services received at KP, not just during this visit" the majority rated it as "very good" or higher, and only a very few rated it as less than "good" (fig. 4.8). Older people and those higher in self-reported social class were most satisfied overall with the care and services. As one elderly respondent said, in summing up her experience, "My doctor takes great interest in me. I've had him a long time. He knows me and knows what

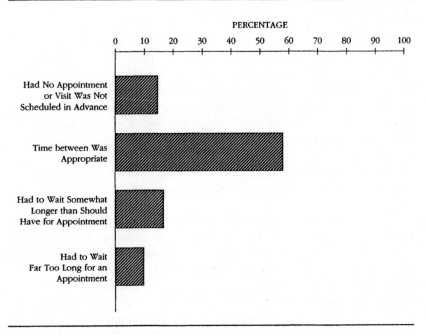

Fig. 4.6. KPNW members' views on the appropriateness of the appointment lag for their most recent office visit.
Source: Data from CHR 1989 Current Membership Survey.

I need. He knows my case; knows how to take care of me. He has my whole history. He's a good doctor."

Overall Satisfaction with KPNW

As part of the 1992 Current Membership Survey, KPNW members, after being asked about their level of satisfaction or dissatisfaction with cost, access, and quality of care and service, were asked about their level of overall satisfaction with KPNW (see fig. 4.5). A great majority reported that they were satisfied or very satisfied. Only a small minority were dissatisfied overall.

In terms of our model, the health attitudes, knowledge, and beliefs that we studied have no effect on overall satisfaction levels. The single best predictor of satisfaction with KPNW overall is satisfaction with overall access to care. Other important predictors are satisfaction with the personal interest of physicians, with the overall cost of care in KPNW, and with the technical competence of the physicians. Demographic and socioeconomic factors are much less important; but being

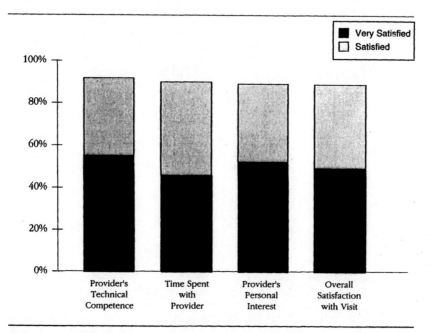

Fig. 4.7. KPNW members' satisfaction with care at their most recent office visit.
Source: Data from CHR 1991 Survey of Medical Office Visits.

older, lower in income and education, and in better health are also predictors of satisfaction (fig. 4.9).

Other Measures of Satisfaction/Dissatisfaction

In addition to being asked to rate their level of satisfaction/dissatisfaction with various aspects of KPNW and its services, KPNW subscribers have routinely been asked in the membership surveys if they and their families have encountered problems in their use of services, what the problems were, and whether they or their families have used services outside of KPNW. The answers to these questions are examined here as behavioral measures of dissatisfaction. Disenrollment is also examined to see to what extent subscribers express dissatisfaction through disenrollment.

PROBLEMS ENCOUNTERED

In our membership surveys, around 20 percent of the respondents reported that they or members of their families had encountered problems in their use of services during the twelve months preceding the survey (fig. 4.10). Though subscribers cite a broad spectrum of problems,

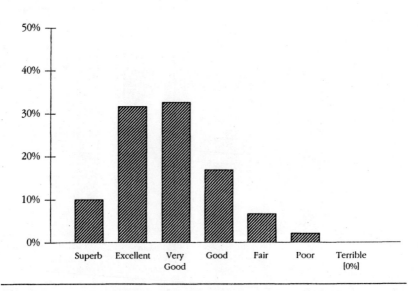

Fig. 4.8. Members' overall rating of care and services at KPNW (not just for their most recent visit).
Source: Data from CHR 1991 Survey of Medical Office Visits.

the most frequently mentioned are related to access, mostly the telephone appointment process and the appointment lag. Less frequently mentioned are problems that have to do with quality of care. These include complaints that something more or something different should have been done, that what was done should have been done sooner, that care was deficient because of something about the medical care system, and the like.

Most of the other problems mentioned had to do with other aspects of the medical care system, including factors that were viewed as inconveniences to patients or as undesirable for some reason (but were not presented as access or quality issues). These include complaints about such things as clinic hours, changes in telephone numbers, the reassignment of personnel from one location to another, the way in which information is communicated inside the system, dealings with the business office (other than claims or coverage problems), and a miscellany of other things characteristic of large organizations.

Problems were more frequently mentioned by subscribers higher in education and income, by younger people, by those making more visits, and by women under age sixty-five.

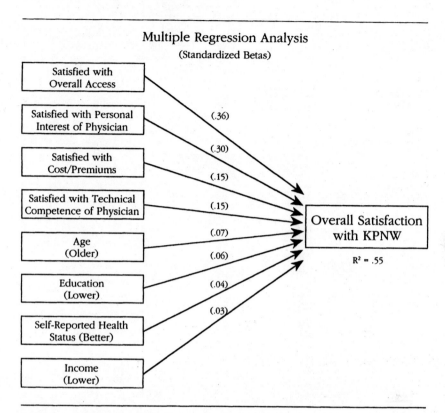

Multiple Regression Analysis
(Standardized Betas)

Satisfied with Overall Access

Satisfied with Personal Interest of Physician (.36)

Satisfied with Cost/Premiums (.30)

Satisfied with Technical Competence of Physician (.15)

Age (Older) (.15)

Education (Lower) (.07)

Self-Reported Health Status (Better) (.06)

Income (Lower) (.04) (.03)

Overall Satisfaction with KPNW
$R^2 = .55$

Fig. 4.9. Significant predictors of overall satisfaction of KPNW subscribers. *Source:* Data from CHR 1985 Current Membership Survey.

THE USE OF OUTSIDE SERVICES

Subscribers have routinely been asked in the membership surveys about their and their families' use of physicians outside KPNW, other than those arranged and paid for through their KPNW coverage (and excluding chiropractors, naturopaths, and others whom some perceive to be physicians). The proportion using outside services has tended to remain fairly constant over the years. As figure 4.11 shows, a small minority of subscribers report using outside services for themselves or someone in their family in the twelve months preceding the survey. The majority of those members who had gone outside reported having made only one visit to an outside physician. The use of outside physicians clearly appears to be episodic rather than routine.

Whereas some use of outside services was to meet a requirement of another organization (e.g., worker's compensation, a life insurance company), was free care or was covered by other insurance or paid for

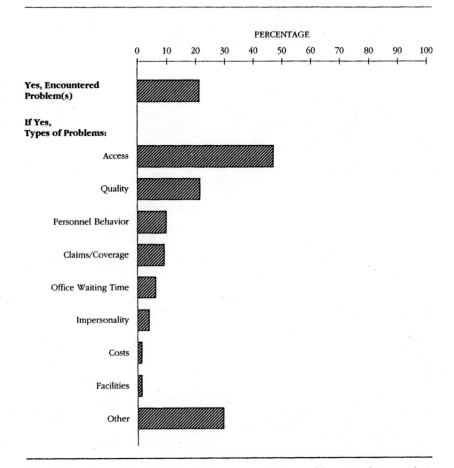

Fig. 4.10. Proportion of subscribers encountering problems in their or their families' use of KPNW services in the last twelve months, and types of problems encountered.

Note: The total of the percentages for "Types of Problem" is greater than 100 percent because more than one type of problem was mentioned.

Source: Data from CHR 1986 Current Membership Survey.

by some other party, or was for a service not covered under KPNW, the primary reason given for using outside services was dissatisfaction with some aspect of KPNW's quality of service or care, or with access— mostly the appointment lag. Much less frequently mentioned were such reasons as the desire to get a second or outside opinion (with no mention of dissatisfaction with KPNW) or the desire to see a former physician or a physician who had been highly recommended by others or whose reputation as a physician was well known in the community. The

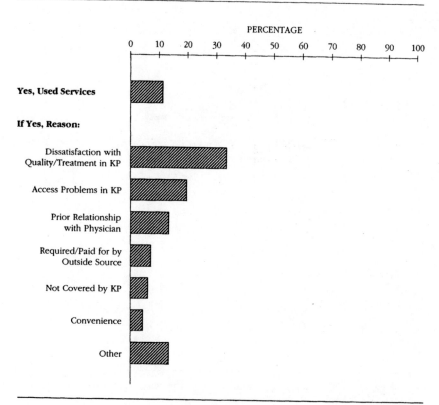

PERCENTAGE

Fig. 4.11. Proportion of KPNW subscribers using non-KPNW services for themselves or their families in the last twelve months and the primary reason for non-KPNW use.
Note: Of those using outside services, 35 percent had all or part paid by other insurance.
Source: Data from CHR 1987 Current Membership Survey.

subscribers using outside services tended to be those higher in income and education, and those who had lived in the area for a greater number of years.

DISENROLLMENT

Over the years, various attempts have been made to find out how much of the disenrollment from KPNW has been because of dissatisfaction, and what the sources of this dissatisfaction have been. We approached this issue by conducting a series of mail questionnaire surveys of random samples of ex-subscribers shortly after they had terminated their KPNW membership. These have been described in earlier work (Pope 1978).

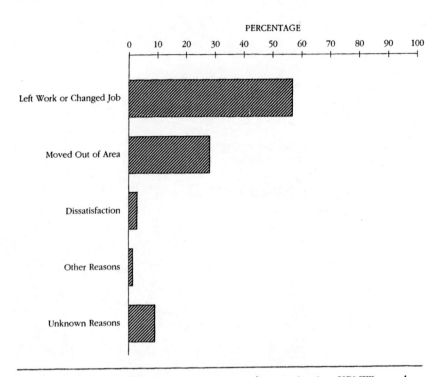

Fig. 4.12. Former subscribers' main reason for terminating KPNW membership.
Source: Data from CHR 1976 Termination Survey.

As figure 4.12 shows, most of the individuals responding to the disenrollment surveys had left the jobs through which they had obtained their KPNW coverage. These included subscribers who had moved out of the area, as well as those who had remained in the area but had changed jobs or left the labor force. Only a small minority of respondents were found to have terminated their membership solely for reasons of dissatisfaction. Most reported themselves to be in excellent or good health, and to have used few services in the year before their termination.

In both the earlier studies and a more recent analysis, the several social and demographic characteristics on which KPNW disenrollees most differ from those not terminating, or from the KPNW membership as a whole, are age, marital status or subscriber unit size, and residency in the service area. Those subscribers terminating membership are disproportionately younger, tend more to be unmarried or one-person subscriber units (i.e., subscribers with no enrolled dependents), and tend to have lived in the geographic area and in their residences for a shorter

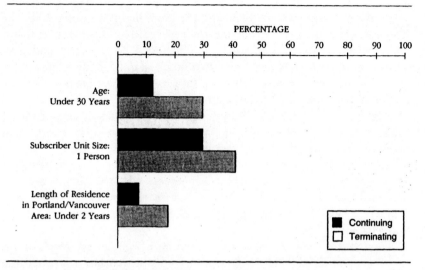

Fig. 4.13. Characteristics of KPNW subscribers terminating their membership between 1985 and 1990, and of those continuing their membership.
Source: Data from CHR 1985 Current Membership Survey, and 1985 and 1990 KP Membership Information Processing System.

time (fig. 4.13). When asked if they would consider again becoming KPNW members (were they to have the opportunity to do so), a majority of those in the termination studies reported that they would. Less than 10 percent said that they definitely would *not* consider it.

Like our findings on satisfaction, our findings on use of outside physicians and on disenrollment are congruent with the research literature. Disenrollment and the use of services outside the HMO plan have been examined as behavioral indicators of dissatisfaction in previous studies (Luft 1981). These are thought to be more objective measures of members' dissatisfaction with managed care. That is to say, they may represent the phenomenon of members "voting with their feet."

Previous studies of other HMOs have found that in any given year some plan members seek care outside the plan even though the services are available within the managed care system and are financially covered by the plan. However, as Donabedian (1969) concluded after summarizing the findings from several different studies, an appreciable proportion of HMO plan members use outside services even though they may be very well satisfied with the care they receive within the system. Both Donabedian (1969) and Weinerman (1964) found that having used a particular physician in the past (e.g., before enrolling in the HMO) was a reason for going outside. From his review, Weinerman found wives of subscribers, long-term members, and the more highly educated to be the heaviest users of services outside their prepaid group practice plans. Other reasons for outside utilization included convenience and easy access. Freidson (1961) concluded that much of outside use relates to lay expectations and the belief that fee-for-service practitioners will more readily accommodate patients' wants.

In general, however, outside services represent a small proportion of the total services received by HMO plan members, and only a very small proportion of members are regular outside users. Dissatisfaction is correlated with outside use, but a relatively small proportion of members are dissatisfied overall. Some HMO members who use outside services may ultimately leave the plan, but not necessarily because of dissatisfaction per se (Weinerman 1964; Pope 1978; Luft 1981; Scitovsky, Benham, and McCall 1981).

Though there is a reasonable amount of published research on enrollment in HMOs, much less published research has addressed the issue of disenrollment (Zapka, Stanek, and Raitt 1986). The study of enrollment and disenrollment conducted in the Health Insurance Plan of Greater New York was the first comprehensive study of disenrollment in an HMO (Densen, Deardorff, and Balamuth 1958). Disenrollment was found to be highest in the first year of enrollment, and retention rates were found to be higher for subscribers with family contracts.

Subsequent studies have reported similar findings—that is, that the probability of disenrollment is highest in the first year after joining and that retention rates tend to be higher for subscribers with dependents and for middle-aged and older subscribers (Forthofer, Glasser, and Light 1979; Mullooly and Freeborn 1979; Luft 1981). Young, one-person subscriber units tend to be overrepresented among those disenrolling (Luft 1981; Wersinger and Sorensen 1982; Boxerman, Hennelly, and Woodward 1984; Wrightson, Genuardi, and Stephens 1987).

No consistent relationships have been found between disenrollment and other social and demographic characteristics such as marital status, sex, race or ethnicity, and the like. The same is also true for health status and the utilization of medical care. Disenrollment because of dissatisfaction with access to care and with the quality of service and care has been characteristic of only a minority of disenrollees. Costs, however, have figured as a significant reason for HMO disenrollment. Studies have shown that consumers are highly sensitive to premium differentials (Piontkowski and Butler 1980; Wintringham 1982) as well as to shifts in their overall share of costs for medical care (Luft 1981; Boxerman, Hennelly, and Woodward 1984).

Findings similar to these have been reported in a recent national poll

(Gallup 1991) that asked enrollees in managed care and traditional plans about their intentions to switch plans. Though slightly more traditional plan enrollees reported that they were likely to change plans at the next open enrollment period, younger enrollees and male subscribers in both types of plans reported this intention more frequently than did older enrollees and female subscribers. The main reasons given (somewhat more frequently by traditional plan enrollees than by managed care enrollees) for possibly switching were cost-related ones—the primary one having to do with premium increases. Price sensitivity to premium increases was found to be very similar for enrollees of both types of plan.

Summary and Discussion

Our findings are generally consistent with previous research on patient satisfaction (Luft 1981; Aharony and Strasser 1993; Williams and Torrens 1993). Overall, a large majority express satisfaction with the KPNW managed care system. However, the level of satisfaction with specific aspects of the program varies considerably. The greatest satisfaction is with cost and coverage and with the technical quality of care. The least satisfaction is with access to care other than emergency care or routine follow-up—that is, care for acute illnesses, including those seen by physicians as self-limiting, and care for conditions the patient may have recognized but accepted or tolerated for some time before deciding to seek care.

The finding that satisfaction is greater when a specific visit is evaluated than when generalizations are made across time and visits is similar to what has been found with regard to people's attitudes toward physicians and practitioners of other professional or higher-level occupations, such as politicians and lawyers. People tend to express rather high levels of dissatisfaction with or distrust of physicians (politicians, lawyers, etc.) in general or as an occupational group, but to be very satisfied with their own physician (representative, senator, lawyer, and so on).

Contrary to what might be inferred from much of the health services literature on managed care and the sociological literature on formal organizations, most KPNW members do not identify physician-patient relationships and lack of concern for patients as individuals (i.e., "impersonality") as significant problems. Although satisfaction levels and perceptions of problems vary somewhat by members' social, economic, and demographic characteristics, and by their health status and use of services, there is much less variation than might be expected.

Dissatisfaction with access to care and with the quality of care or service in KPNW were important reasons—although not the only reasons—for using outside services. But even so, most episodes of outside care consisted of a single visit. Dissatisfaction per se plays a relatively small role in disenrollment. Members disenroll mainly because of job changes or loss of employment, or because they move out of the area. Relatively few (though the number is significant over time) leave solely because of dissatisfaction.

In sum, though members are not satisfied with all aspects of KPNW, and many report that they have encountered problems with KPNW, their dissatisfactions are balanced, according to their own reports, by the advantages they believe KPNW offers in the way of lower costs, comprehensiveness of coverage, the absence of paperwork (e.g., no insurance forms), and access to a generally high quality of care when it is "really needed."

We began this chapter by noting that patient satisfaction is an important, and often neglected, element in the appraisal of managed care. That the customer is generally happy, however, does not conclusively argue that the product is sound. At least as important is the judgment of those who provide the care and who, at one level at least, are more qualified to evaluate the success of the prepaid group practice model of managed care as a social enterprise. Having asked the patient, therefore, we need also to ask the physician.

5

Physician Satisfaction with Managed Care

> Not all that enhances rationality
> reduces happiness, and not all that increases
> happiness reduces efficiency.
> —Amitai Etzioni

The future success of HMOs as a national strategy largely depends on their ability to recruit and keep qualified physicians. Physician satisfaction with the work setting is an essential element in the effectiveness of managed care since high levels of dissatisfaction may affect both turnover rates and the quality of care (Luft 1981; Mick et al. 1983; Lichtenstein 1984a; Lichtenstein 1984b). Physician satisfaction can also influence patient satisfaction, which has consequences for membership retention in managed care plans (Mechanic 1975; Linn et al. 1985). As Lichtenstein pointed out, "the task of retaining physicians is a crucial one not only because the organization must maintain its own stability and predictability, but also because the organization must seek to maintain the stability of the doctor-patient relationship and the continuity of care provided by physicians to patients" (Lichtenstein 1984b, 166). Physician satisfaction is a prerequisite for the growth of HMOs, and the inability to recruit enough qualified physicians may be more of a limiting factor to managed care than the inability to attract patients (Luft 1981). In this chapter, we focus on how a prepaid group practice HMO affects the job satisfaction of physicians and how physicians view their experiences in practicing in this type of setting.

HMOs are thought to offer many advantages for physicians, such as the opportunity to provide high-quality care and to concentrate on professional functions and patients' needs rather than the business aspects of practice. Other reported advantages include regular and predictable working hours, reasonable incomes relative to work loads, fewer night calls and longer vacations, access to colleagues for consultations, and opportunities for continuing education and professional development. Nevertheless, many physicians are skeptical about managed care and fear that the growth of HMOs will decrease professional autonomy, reduce physician incomes, and result in a poorer quality of care (Scheckler and Schulz 1987; Schulz et al. 1990; Berenson 1991; Iglehart 1992a). Managed care may also lead to increasing conflicts between physicians and management (Madison and Konrad 1988; Astrachan and Astrachan 1989). This is because of medicine being what Freidson (1970) called a "dominant profession."

Freidson (1970) distinguished dominant professions from other occupational groups and argued that medicine is the foremost example of a dominant profession. Through legal means and public approval, members of the medical profession have gained the right to control medical work and to have autonomy in clinical decisions (Starr 1982). The medical profession has a monopoly over the content of its work, and attempts by those outside of the profession to control or evaluate medical work are officially illegitimate. Freidson called this "organized autonomy," which he considered the single most distinctive feature of a true profession. Other occupational groups in the health field share many of the values and attributes of a profession, but they do not have "organized autonomy." For the most part, medicine defines and controls the core content of the work of most other health occupations and therefore dominates the medical hierarchy. No other members of the health care team have this level of power and autonomy. Although medicine has seen some erosion in its autonomy and control in recent years, Freidson argued that medicine will continue to control the core content of its work and will maintain its basic dominance for years to come. Control over the allocation of resources to health care, however, will be seriously contested by managers, policy makers, and politicians. Physicians may no longer be able to dominate these types of decisions (Freidson 1985).

The literature on formal organizations has assumed that professionals and bureaucratic organizations are inherently antagonistic because bureaucratic characteristics conflict with basic professional values and principles of organization (Scott 1966; Lichtenstein 1984b). A long-standing premise about professionals, such as physicians, in bureaucratic organizations is that they have a set of internalized standards and norms to guide their practice and that these may conflict with the patterns of individual behavior required for organizational effectiveness (Parsons 1951; Scott 1966). Bureaucratic values emphasize corporate responsibility, adherence to organizational rules and procedures, service and loyalty to the organization and its goals, and submission to authority based on formally defined hierarchical positions. In contrast, professional values emphasize the autonomy and responsibility of the individual practitioner, service to the client, loyalty to colleagues, and allegiance to collegial authority based on competency and expertise (Hall 1977; Coe 1978).

Freidson (1970), however, distinguished between control over the core content of physicians' work and control over the social and economic conditions of work. The content of physicians' work falls under the protection of organized autonomy, but control over the social and economic aspects of practice is not protected. This distinction is not always recognized by physicians (or managers) and can lead to conflicts when physicians work in formal organizations. Concerns about autonomy and professional prerogatives often grow out of this ambiguity regarding which areas of work should be under professional control and which are the legitimate domain of management. Control over the content of work and the organization of the work environment are major concerns for physicians, and how this problem is worked out plays a large role in physician job satisfaction as well as in the effectiveness of managed care systems (Lichtenstein 1984b; Greenlick 1989).

Conflict is not inevitable, however, and too little attention has been paid to the accommodation of organizations to professionals. Through various mechanisms, professionals can create their own organizational structures within the larger organization. In reality, the relationship is interactive and characterized by influence running in both directions: organizations influence professionals, but professionals also modify organizations. Powerful professional groups, such as physicians, can often force health care organizations to change their structures to satisfy professional needs (Lichtenstein 1984b; Smith and Kaluzny 1986).

Most hospitals and health care systems have a dual authority structure with a medical hierarchy separate from the formal administrative hierarchy (Shortell and Kaluzny 1988; Shortell 1991). This type of structure helps ameliorate professional-organizational conflict, and physicians have created mechanisms through which organizational needs can be accommodated without compromising physicians' professional norms and values (Goss 1961; Freidson 1975). The contention that bureaucratization and professionalism are inherently in conflict may be overstated. Although professionals resist organizational mechanisms that encroach on autonomy, certain bureaucratic characteristics can enhance the work of professionals. Clear lines of authority and responsibility, formal rules and standard operating procedures, mechanisms that promote coordination of activities and effective communication, skilled support personnel, and modern equipment and facilities are attributes of organizations that can facilitate professional work and improve its efficiency. Organizations can provide resources and facilities that may not be readily available to individual professionals. In medicine, many technical resources are available only in formal organizations such as large hospitals and HMOs. If organizations facilitate access to resources and coordinate activities in ways that do not interfere with the core content of professional work, they are likely to be accepted by professionals (Hall 1977; Lichtenstein 1984b).

In recent years these ideas have increasingly been expressed in the health services and management literature as the conflict between two cultures—the culture of professionals, represented particularly by physicians, and the culture of management (or business). Greenlick (1989) argued that the differences in culture between physicians and managers must be better understood if the health care system is to function more effectively. Physician leaders and HMO managers must mediate the conflict between the two cultures and socialize physicians to the values and norms of managed care while at the same time socializing managers to the values and norms of medicine. That is to say, this process is not a one-way street. The resolution of these sources of conflict may be the single most important function of managers and physician leaders in managed care settings.

A principal concern has been that managed care will place physicians in roles that seriously conflict with their professional values. This situation could lead to high levels of physician dissatisfaction, since physicians may perceive that they have to practice in ways that are incompatible with their internalized values (Schmoldt 1991). Ultimately, this problem could make managed care settings unstable and compromise their effectiveness. It becomes important, therefore, to identify potential sources of conflict and strain for physicians in managed care systems in order to find ways to avoid conflict and to ameliorate serious problems (Lichtenstein 1984b; Greenlick 1989).

As might be expected from the above discussion, much of the research on physicians in managed care settings has dealt with the question, Does the type of practice setting affect the job satisfaction of physicians? Several early studies found that physicians in small fee-for-service groups and solo practices were more satisfied overall than were physicians in more bureaucratic settings (e.g., large publicly operated systems and prepaid groups). Constraints on autonomy and conflicts over income distribution appeared to be the most important sources of dissatisfaction among physicians in these settings (Ben-David 1958; McElrath 1961; Ross 1969; Donabedian 1969; Prybil 1971; Mechanic 1972; Mechanic 1975). Most of these studies compared large prepaid group practices with traditional fee-for-service practice and were not able to separate the effects of how physicians were paid from the effects of how care was organized (Lichtenstein 1984b). Research on physician satisfaction in other managed care settings, such as IPAs and PPOs, has been very limited (Rosko and Broyles 1988).

The underlying source of physician dissatisfaction may be the sense of a lack of control over the work environment and not management interference with professional autonomy and patient care decisions. Several studies report that physicians in HMO settings are less satisfied than are fee-for-service physicians with their control over the pace of work, patient load, scheduling, the time they can spend with patients, and other aspects of the practice environment (Mechanic 1976; Astrachan and Astrachan 1989). Luft's 1981 review of physician satisfaction in HMOs concluded that HMO physicians were satisfied with most aspects of practice and felt that they could practice good medicine in the HMO setting. Few were unhappy with their incomes and working hours. Some problems remained, however. According to Luft, these derive from

> a combination of minimal incentives to expand hours, the resultant overwhelming patient load, the lack of medically interesting cases, and a loss of control. When faced with increases in patient demand, the salaried physician has no incentive, except genuine concern, to work longer hours. However, HMO patients are less likely to know when their physician is working overtime and are less appreciative. They cannot be consistently shuffled off to someone else because of the plan's responsibilities to treat enrollees. Overworked physicians do not have enough time to devote to their patients, and this often means that psychosocial problems are treated symptomatically. This is frustrating for the physician who is trained to cure rare diseases, rather than deal with such problems as alcoholism, stress, and poor diet. Such major problems are labeled trivial, rather than recognized as areas in which traditional medical care breaks down. (Luft 1981, 318)

Several studies (Mechanic 1972; Freidson 1973; Mechanic 1975; Barr 1983) have reported that physician-patient interactions can be a source of dissatisfaction for physicians practicing in HMOs. Patients are more likely to be seen as neurotic or overly demanding, as seeking care for minor or trivial problems, as prone to "shop around from doctor to doctor," and so on. Mechanic (1972) found that these problems were more a reflection of the physicians' general dissatisfaction than of patients' actual behavior. Most ambulatory care patients in both HMOs and traditional settings are not seriously ill (Mechanic 1975). These patient problems may be overstated. Physicians' responses may be unduly weighted by a few cases or by unpleasant incidents (Darsky, Sinai, and Axelrod 1958; Luft 1981; Freeborn 1985). Physicians' views have been found to vary by specialty, in that patient-related problems are perceived to be greater by adult primary care physicians—the "gate-keepers" in HMOs (Barr 1983).

Within managed care plans, physician satisfaction levels have been found to vary by age, participation in decision making, and specialty (Mechanic 1975; Barr and Steinberg 1983; Lichtenstein 1984a). Recent studies show that practicing in managed care is not uniformly associated with lower levels of satisfaction and that the advantages of practice in managed care settings may be perceived to outweigh the disadvantages (Schulz et al. 1990; Baker and Cantor 1993).

Reports of serious conflicts between physicians and managers are rare. Conflicts are greater, however, in those organizational situations where professionals are least likely to be able to structure their own work (Lichtenstein 1984b). For example, in some staff-model HMOs major conflicts have arisen between physicians and HMO management. In this type of HMO, physicians are employees, and physician managers are integrated into the overall management structure of the HMO. In this situation, erosion of professional authority and control may be more likely.

The group-model HMO provides an example of an organizational arrangement that attempts to accommodate physicians' needs for autonomy and self-regulation within a highly formalized organizational structure. In this model, the medical group is an independent professional corporation governed by the physicians. This structure permits the physicians to exercise internal control of their affairs and to maintain jurisdiction over their professional activities. Peer review and self-regulation are inherent in this form of organization, and formal control over the quality of care and the content of medical work remains with the physicians. The physicians are not under the formal administrative hierarchy of the managed care plan. This dual authority structure does not totally mitigate conflict, however. Many gray areas remain, and the issue of professional versus administrative authority can still be problematic.

Our Findings

Our studies of physician satisfaction are based on questionnaire surveys of the physicians comprising Northwest Permanente (NWP). NWP is the independent medical group that contracts exclusively with the Kaiser Foundation Health Plan of the Northwest to provide or arrange for all professional medical services to Kaiser Foundation Health Plan members at an agreed-upon capitation rate—that is, a rate per member per month—that is established prospectively each year. The NWP physician surveys were conducted in 1977, 1984, and 1991, but we focus here mostly on data from the most recent survey (which had an 84% response rate). In each survey, the questionnaires were self-administered and took about two hours to complete. The basic content of the questionnaires was similar over time, but some new sections were added in 1991 to reflect new concerns and issues. In general, respondents and non-respondents were similar on basic background characteristics, particularly in 1991. (Further details on the surveys and research methods are provided in the Appendix, below.)

In the following section, we describe the background characteristics of the physicians and their reasons for joining NWP. We then describe the physicians' views on and evaluations of their experiences with practicing in this setting, their views as to what are the advantages and disadvantages of KPNW, and their satisfaction/dissatisfaction with specific aspects of their work. The next section compares the satisfaction of primary care physicians with that of other physicians. The final section deals with factors influencing overall satisfaction.

Figure 5.1 presents our framework for thinking about the determinants of physician satisfaction and the way in which physician satisfaction relates to organizational effectiveness. Our model draws heavily upon the work of Karasek and Theorell (1990), who hypothesized that job satisfaction in most settings is primarily a function of work demands, decision latitude, skill use, and social supports. Jobs characterized by heavy psychological demands, limited decision latitude, limited use of skills, and limited social supports are the most stressful and produce the most dissatisfaction. This job situation also increases mental strain and may cause physical illness (Karasek 1979).

The Physician in KPNW

Information on the background of NWP physicians is given in figure 5.2. Most of the physicians in the medical group are board certified in their specialties: a higher percentage of NWP physicians than of physicians in the local community are board certified. NWP physicians have traditionally been trained in some of the most prestigious medical schools in the nation, and the KPNW medical care program is fully accredited by all the major national accreditation agencies. Many of the physicians (one out of four) also hold teaching appointments at the Oregon Health Sciences University School of Medicine (the state's only medical school). NWP offers a residency program in conjunction with this institution.

Foreign medical graduates have consistently represented less than 10

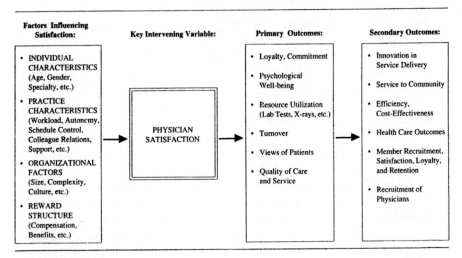

Fig. 5.1. The importance of physician satisfaction to organizational effectiveness (hypothesized relationships).

percent of NWP physicians. This figure is similar to the proportion of foreign medical graduates in the local medical community. Although most NWP physicians are male, the proportion of women physicians in NWP has steadily increased and is somewhat higher than that in the U.S. medical profession as a whole. The most frequent category of prior practice experience is residency training; this reflects the percentage of physicians who are under forty years of age.

The assumption that managed care organizations employ inferior and poorly trained physicians is not supported by our data or by the findings of other studies (Luft 1988; Rosko and Broyles 1988). Background information on NWP physicians suggests that they are highly qualified.

Reasons for Joining NWP

In our surveys, physicians were provided a list of possible reasons for choosing this practice setting and were asked to indicate the importance of each reason. The major reasons given for joining were, in order of importance, the community and its quality of life, the desire for regular working hours, the desire to avoid problems of office management, the desire for stable and predictable income and benefits, and the desire to be able to provide care without having to consider the cost to the patient. Opportunities to work with peers and the opportunity to provide high-quality medical care were also ranked fairly highly (fig. 5.3). We also asked the physicians to tell us what they considered to be the two or

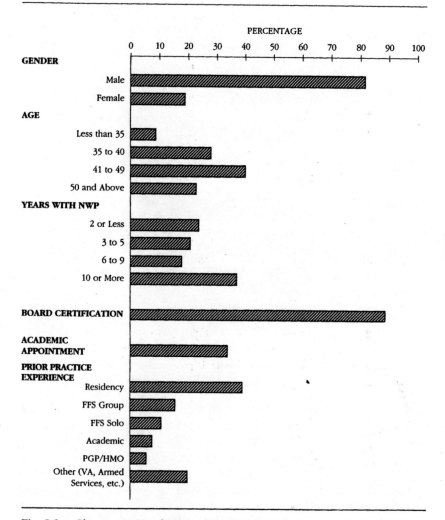

Fig. 5.2. Characteristics of NWP physicians. *FFS*, fee-for-service; *PGP*, prepaid group practice; *VA*, Veterans' Administration.
Source: Data from CHR 1991 Survey of NWP Physicians.

three most significant advantages of practicing in this setting. The most frequently mentioned advantage was less pressure, as reflected in such features as regular working hours, night and weekend coverage, and so on. The second most frequently mentioned advantage was freedom from office management and from the business aspects of practice.

Our findings are consistent with those of other studies. Regular working hours and more leisure time, freedom from the problems of office

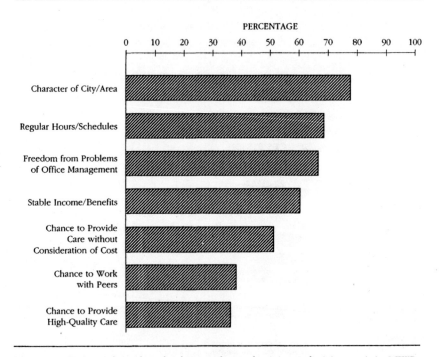

Fig. 5.3. Factors that played a large role in physicians' decision to join NWP. *Source:* Data from CHR 1991 Survey of NWP Physicians.

management, the ability to provide care without having to consider the cost to the patient, stable incomes and benefits, access to colleagues, and the like have been often reported as the major desiderata that physicians cite in explaining their decision to join HMOs (Luft 1981; Budrys 1993). Wolinsky (1982) analyzed data from a national survey of forty-five hundred physicians and compared physicians in solo practice, small group practice, and large group practice. Those opting for large group practices were more likely to be younger and board certified. Physicians opting for large group practices also tended to be motivated more by professional factors, such as quality of medical care and opportunities for professional contacts. For these physicians, personal autonomy and income potential played less of a role in determining choice of practice than they did for other physicians. Autonomy and income were of primary importance to the physicians who chose traditional solo practice and small group practice.

Luft (1981) pointed out that physicians have a number of attractive practice alternatives, including traditional fee-for-service practice. Satisfaction can be viewed as a continuum ranging from preference, to satisfaction, to dissatisfaction, to rejection. When considering physicians' satisfaction with prepaid group practice, one must keep in mind that the HMO managed care option is something that physicians choose—it is not imposed on them—and that those who select it may be different from those who choose traditional practice. For example, the non-entrepreneurial physician may be more inclined to select an HMO-type practice. Or it may be that physicians who choose HMOs are less concerned with autonomy and more concerned with predictability of working hours and reasonable work loads. In other words, it is possible that only those physicians who like the concept of prepaid group practice enter HMOs in the first place, which in turn may make them more likely to be satisfied with the setting. By definition, surveys of HMO physicians leave out physicians who have rejected the HMO model (for whatever reasons), and this situation applies to our data as well. This needs to be kept in mind in the sections that follow.

Luft also emphasized that the transition from one form of practice to another is very difficult and costly, both financially and psychologically. Low turnover rates among HMO physicians seem to support this assumption (Lichtenstein 1984b). These low turnover rates may also reflect the fact that physicians find HMOs to be a satisfying practice alternative. However, as Luft noted, the difficulty of moving from one form of practice to another may cause HMO physicians to express their dissatisfaction by trying to change the system rather than by leaving it and having to start all over again (Luft 1981).

Physicians' Views about Practicing in KPNW

Our surveys show that most NWP physicians would choose this setting again, given the choice, and most were satisfied with their careers. The majority were satisfied with their current income and with their work load. Almost all felt that their relations with their colleagues were positive and that the quality of care in KPNW was very good or excellent (fig. 5.4). Earlier, we indicated that many community physicians fear that HMOs provide poor-quality care. In contrast, our findings show that NWP physicians consider the technical quality of care in this setting to be equal to or better than that provided in the community. These findings on quality are reinforced by empirical studies that show that the large prepaid group practice HMOs provide care that is of high quality and comparable to that provided in other settings (Cunningham and Williamson 1980; Luft 1988; Rosko and Broyles 1988).

In contrast to the impression given in much of the professional literature, most NWP physicians do not perceive that practicing in KPNW

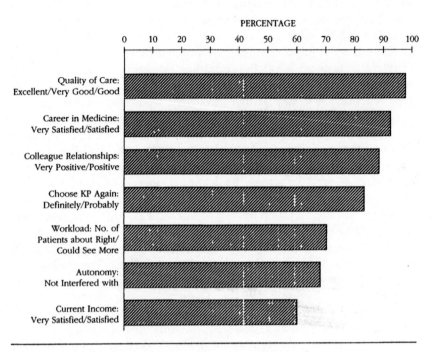

Fig. 5.4. NWP physicians' attitudes about selected aspects of practice in KPNW.
Source: Data from CHR 1991 Survey of NWP Physicians.

seriously limits their professional autonomy and freedom. Of the minority who indicate that KPNW attempts to influence their use of resources to a large extent, most report that this influence is fair and reasonable. Because of the importance of the topic of professional autonomy in the literature, we asked physicians about the extent to which KPNW attempted to influence various aspects of practice, including the use of laboratory and imaging procedures (e.g., x-rays), referral and prescribing decisions, and hospital admissions (fig. 5.5). Except in the case of external referrals, most of the survey respondents did not feel that KPNW interfered with their use of resources. Eighty-seven percent agreed with the statement "I have the freedom and support to make important clinical decisions."

Freidson's early studies of prepaid group practice also suggested that infringement on professional autonomy was not a major issue. Exercise of control (either by other physicians or by physician management) over

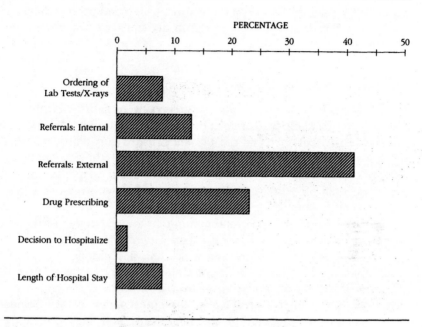

Fig. 5.5. NWP physicians reporting that KPNW attempts to influence physicians' use of resources "to a large extent" in certain areas.
Source: Data from CHR 1991 Survey of NWP Physicians.

HMO physicians' medical decisions and practice patterns was limited. In most cases, peer review and formal evaluation of physicians' clinical work were lacking. In fact, most of the physicians included in the study had only limited information on the practices of other physicians outside of their own department (Freidson 1975). After a thorough review of the literature on this issue, Luft concluded: "The weight of evidence suggests that the autonomy issue is largely a non-problem. While physicians still value autonomy, they reluctantly accept numerous restrictions, and they often find organizations helpful. Group practices seem to offer valuable clinical supports that are seen to be necessary for good practice" (Luft 1981, 313).

A recent national survey of young physicians examined the association between practicing in managed care and the levels of perceived professional autonomy (Baker and Cantor 1993). Managed care practice was related to lower levels of perceived autonomy in patient selection and time allocation but to higher levels of autonomy in medical decision making and the use of resources. HMO management decisions, such as cost-quality trade-offs on capital investment, imposed practice limits on physicians, but these resource allocation decisions are not made at the individual level.

Satisfaction with Specific Aspects of Practice

Most respondents to the physician surveys were satisfied with their working hours, their patient relationships, the continuity of care, the number of new patients, and the amount of extra duty. Participation in decisions affecting work life, schedule control, and ability to influence the work environment were more problematic for these physicians (fig. 5.6). Less than 50 percent of them were satisfied with these last three aspects of their practice.

These results reinforce the assumption that the underlying issues may be a sense of lack of control over the work environment and resources—and not management interference with clinical decisions and patient care. Dissatisfaction seems to derive mainly from problems relating to allocation of resources and control over how work is structured and organized (see below). Control over the core content of professional work remains the domain of the physicians, and infringement on professional autonomy is not the chief concern.

Views of How KPNW Compares to Other Plans

We asked NWP physicians the following question: "When asked, do you recommend that people enroll in Kaiser Permanente?" The vast majority of the physicians indicated that they do recommend that persons should enroll.

We also asked the physicians to give their opinions on how the KPNW program's advantages for patients compare with those of other health plans (fig. 5.7). Almost all of the physicians felt that KPNW provided equal or more benefits at a lower premium. Most also felt that KPNW provided better-quality care than did traditional plans and made it easier for patients to see appropriate providers. Another perceived advantage was the availability of medical care when people really need it (e.g., for acute problems and emergency care). A majority of the respondents also noted that KPNW members did not have to spend time doing paperwork and filling out claims and other forms to receive benefits—a major complaint of members (and physicians) about most other plans. The convenience and attractiveness of facilities and shorter waiting times in the medical offices were also often viewed as advantages.

The major disadvantages for KPNW members, according to the phy-

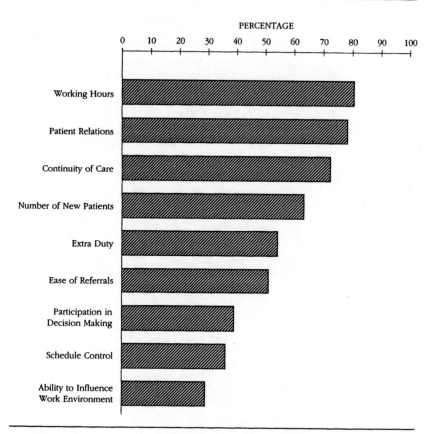

PERCENTAGE

Fig. 5.6. NWP physicians "very satisfied" or "satisfied" with various aspects of practice.
Source: Data from CHR 1991 Survey of NWP Physicians.

sicians, were problems with access for routine care and choice of physician. Most felt that getting a non-emergency appointment with a physician was more difficult in KPNW than in other health plans. Many physicians also felt that KPNW made it more difficult for persons to have a regular physician or to see the same physician most of the time (although, as shown in chapter 3, most KPNW members report that they have a regular physician).

Specialty and Satisfaction

Many of the issues mentioned above are likely to be affected by the different conditions of practice faced by various kinds of specialists, and

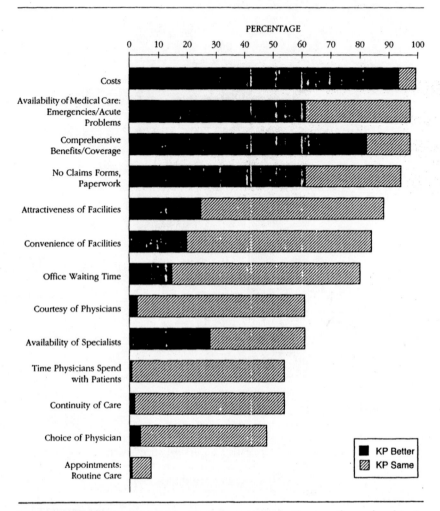

Fig. 5.7. NWP physicians' views on how the advantages of membership in KPNW compared to those of membership in other plans.
Note: Not shown is the percentage who selected the "not as good" response.
Source: Data from CHR 1984 Survey of NWP Physicians.

several studies suggest that managed care may be more problematic for primary care physicians, such as general internists and family physicians (Mechanic 1972; Mechanic 1975; Barr 1983; Baker and Cantor 1993). Our findings only partially support this assumption. Primary care physicians (internists and family physicians), pediatricians, and medical subspecialists were more likely than most other specialists to say that

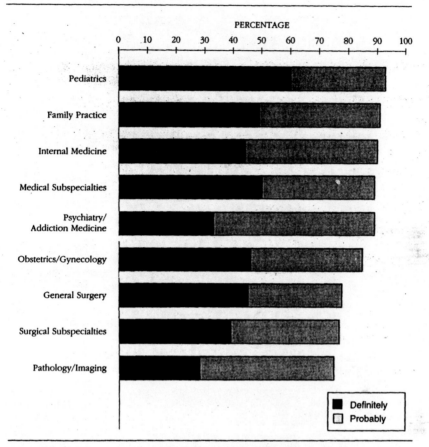

Fig. 5.8. NWP physicians' overall satisfaction (the proportion of those in various specialties who would "probably" or "definitely" choose KPNW again). *Source:* Data from CHR 1991 Survey of NWP Physicians.

they would choose the KPNW setting again (fig. 5.8). Primary care physicians were also more satisfied with the income and fringe benefits they were receiving. However, they were less satisfied than other specialists with most other aspects of practice, including their work load, the number of new patients, schedule control, ease of referrals, and time with patients (fig. 5.9).

As mentioned earlier, problems with patients and physician-patient relationships have been reported as major sources of dissatisfaction for physicians in managed care, particularly primary care physicians. These do not appear to be significant concerns for physicians in NWP (fig.

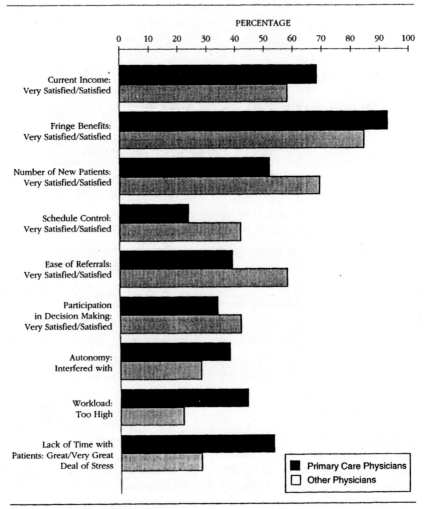

PERCENTAGE

Fig. 5.9. NWP physicians' attitudes about selected aspects of practice in KPNW.
Source: Data from CHR 1991 Survey of NWP Physicians.

5.10). For example, patients overconcerned with minor symptoms, demanding or neurotic patients, and patients shopping around from physician to physician were not considered troublesome problems by the majority of NWP physicians (whether primary care physicians or other specialists). An exception was lack of compliance with medical advice regarding diet, smoking, alcohol use, and other health practices. More than 50 percent of the primary care physicians considered this to be a

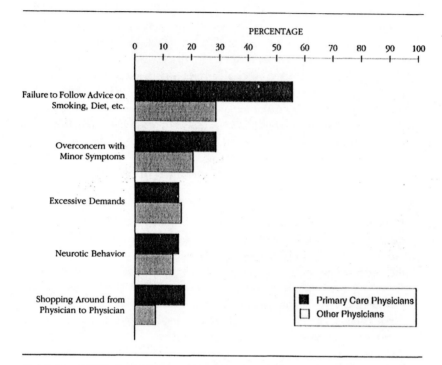

Fig. 5.10. NWP physicians reporting various problems with patients as "troublesome."
Source: Data from CHR 1991 Survey of NWP Physicians.

troublesome issue. Frustration with this problem is widespread among physicians, regardless of the setting. It probably reflects physicians' inability and lack of training to deal with these kinds of complex behavior problems (Mechanic 1972; Mechanic 1975).

General internists and family physicians provide the bulk of adult primary care in the KPNW setting and are the "gatekeepers." This role can be in conflict with physicians' professional values and norms about how they should practice (Katz 1992). Primary care physicians tend to have heavy work loads and fairly rigid appointment schedules (which influence their perceptions about the adequacy of the time they can spend with each patient). They are expected to meet patients' needs and, at the same time, conserve resources and meet other organizational objectives. This situation can be frustrating and contributes to a sense of loss of control for primary care physicians. Some primary care physicians also feel that their contributions are undervalued. As one primary care physician put it:

I think that we primary care physicians are undervalued. Some of us like coordinating care and acting as a liaison. I also think the territory we cover in primary care is too vast to really do justice to the panel sizes we are assigned. If we are asked to do Paps, and other prevention, cover acute and chronic problems, and deal with psychosocial issues—we need more time. The primary care physician's major tool is time. We don't need gismos and gadgets like the radiologists, surgeons, and cardiologists. We need time to explain things to patients.

Another primary care physician commented on the failure to recognize the value of primary care.

I would like to see the medical group improve life for the front-line doctors. Realizing the inequities between specialist and primary care is the beginning. Primary care needs to be supported as an important part of the total system, the role that it plays needs to be defined better. This new definition should be something that all internists can be proud of as well as other primary providers. Compensation for all hours worked is important, too, but I feel [it] is not as important as recognition from the medical group of the value of the primary care provider.

Time pressure and sense of lack of control are reflected in this comment: "The major frustration I have at KP is the expectation to see an unreasonably large number of patients in an unreasonably short period of time. This creates a demand for efficiency at the expense of thoroughness and the ability to teach the patient what they want to know."

To keep these findings in perspective, we need to remember that most of the primary care physicians would choose this setting again and were generally satisfied with working in KPNW. That is to say, the advantages of practice in this setting considerably outweighed the disadvantages.

One primary care physician expressed it this way:

First and foremost, if being a physician is ever going to be a job, then this is the way to do it. The patients who choose KP are reasonable about seeing a variety of providers (both MD and allied health). The physicians work reasonably well together (nothing is perfect, especially considering the personality type that becomes a physician). The schedule in the clinic, while packed and hectic most days, comes to a predictable scheduled end. Evening events can be scheduled and reliably attended. We do QA [quality assurance] in a group setting with as little as possible threat (again this is never going to be perfect) to our individual credibility. We learn from our mistakes. We do not feel competitive towards each other as in the private practice setting and we enthusiastically share learning across departments. Patients are saved the cost and inconvenience of subspecialty consultation when the primary care doctor can just pick up the phone or inter-office mail the chart to the subspecialist for an opinion. In sum, there is much to be thankful for working for this medical group, and I know [this] after spending years in the private practice world. There are many other benefits that I don't have the time to enumerate.

In our surveys, we did not directly ask NWP physicians about their views of the gatekeeping function. One recent study in an HMO setting (Budrys 1993) specifically addressed this issue and found that primary care physicians supported the concept and were committed to gatekeeping. They complained, however, about the frustrations associated with this role, particularly when it came into conflict with their need for mutually satisfying physician-patient relationships. Not surprisingly, surgeons and subspecialists also strongly supported the gatekeeping concept because it allowed them to see only those patients who needed to see them and permitted them to restrict their practices to what they were professionally trained to do. In general, the gatekeeping arrangements allowed the non–primary care specialists to provide high-quality care and freed them from the economic and social pressures of having to cultivate a referral network.

Predictors of Overall Satisfaction

More than 70 percent of the respondents to the physician surveys agreed with the statement "I am extremely glad that I chose this organization to work for over others I was considering at the time I joined." When we asked physicians whether, if they could choose all over again, they would choose KPNW as a place to practice, only 5 percent said that they would not choose this setting again.

What characteristics distinguish those physicians who would choose this setting again from those who would not? Gender did not affect overall satisfaction, but age was important: older physicians were more likely to indicate that they would definitely choose this practice setting again (fig. 5.11). As we saw earlier, specialty also affected overall satisfaction. Pediatricians and medical subspecialists were the most likely to indicate that they would definitely choose this setting again, although most physicians in each specialty said that they would probably choose KPNW again, given the choice (fig. 5.8).

In terms of our model, the most important predictors of overall

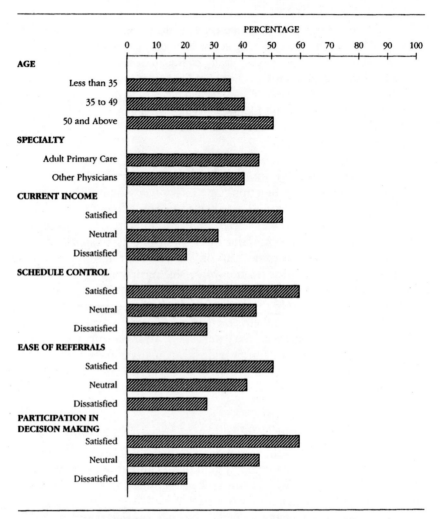

Fig. 5.11. The proportion of NWP physicians who would "definitely" choose KPNW again, by age, speciality, and level of satisfaction.
Source: Data from CHR 1991 Survey of NWP Physicians.

satisfaction were satisfaction with participation in decision making, satisfaction with income, and satisfaction with schedule control. Other significant factors were specialty, ease of referrals, and autonomy (fig. 5.12). Physicians who were satisfied with these aspects of practice were more satisfied overall. When we limited the analysis to only primary care physicians, the findings were similar (except for income). These findings, which appear to be congruent with the assumptions of Karasek and

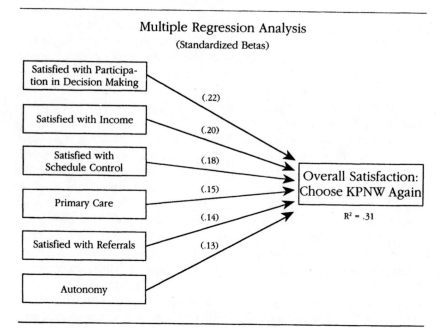

Fig. 5.12. Significant predictors of overall satisfaction among NWP physicians.
Source: Data from CHR 1991 Survey of NWP Physicians.

Theorell (1990), provide further evidence that physicians' major concern is participation in decisions affecting their work life and their control of the work environment—not interference with clinical decisions and the technical quality of care.

Summary and Discussion

Although many community physicians are skeptical about managed care, our findings, as well as those of other studies, suggest that at least the prepaid group practice HMO model of managed care has many advantages for physicians. Most NWP physicians in our surveys were satisfied with their careers and with most aspects of practice in this setting. The vast majority would choose this practice setting again, given the choice. NWP physicians would also recommend this form of practice to other physicians and this form of health plan to lay people who are not currently HMO members.

Professional autonomy was not a major concern for most NWP physicians, and the quality of care at KPNW was considered to be equal to or better than that provided in the community. The physicians viewed their income and benefits favorably, and most felt that the general pressures of practice were reasonable. Perhaps the most important advantage for physicians is that an HMO allows a work schedule with fewer night calls and longer vacations. The increased leisure time growing out of a more flexible schedule and relief from patient care responsibilities allows the physician to lead a more balanced life, with time for self or family.

In the past, lack of acceptance by community physicians was a source of dissatisfaction for physicians in HMOs, particularly prepaid group practices (Luft 1981). This situation made it difficult to recruit highly qualified physicians in some areas (particularly in specialties in short supply, such as orthopedics). This finding also reflects the history of prepaid plans, which were initially viewed as a deviant form of practice by organized medicine. More recent studies suggest that this issue is no longer a significant problem and that physicians who work in HMOs are generally accepted by community physicians (Luft 1981; Lichtenstein 1984a; Freeborn 1985). In recent years, NWP has been able to recruit highly qualified specialists in all areas, which adds to the stature of the medical group and enhances the availability of well-trained colleagues for consultations and referrals. Physician-patient ratios at KPNW are more favorable now than in the past, and there have been substantial additions of new types of personnel, such as physician assistants and nurse practitioners.

Our findings show that physicians and patients have similar views regarding the advantages and disadvantages of KPNW. Both groups perceive that KPNW offers major advantages in terms of price and comprehensive benefits and access to care when you really need it. Both patients and physicians see the lack of hassle regarding forms, paperwork, and the like as a major advantage. The availability of specialty care, the high quality of care, and convenient facilities are other advantages that are recognized by both groups.

The views of the two groups also seem congruent regarding the disadvantages of the HMO setting. Both physicians and patients view access to routine care and continuity of care as problematic, and both express frustration regarding various "bureaucratic" aspects of managed care—such as the difficulty of getting through the system to talk with a physician, and of getting a non-emergency appointment. Patients' and physicians' views reflect the reality that different types of health plans have both advantages and disadvantages. Their views also reflect underlying differences between the organizational features of prepaid group practice HMOs and those of fee-for-service plans. In any setting, patients and physicians have to make trade-offs.

Although we found that most NWP physicians are satisfied with their HMO setting, much of the health services literature still gives the impression that managed care will significantly increase physician dissatisfaction and lead to growing conflicts between physicians and managers. Many physicians also continue to be skeptical about this form of practice. A national opinion poll showed that from 1981 to 1984 the percentage of U.S. physicians reporting at least a somewhat favorable attitude toward HMOs increased from 36 percent to 50 percent (Louis Harris and Associates 1985), and a recent national survey of young physicians showed that the move toward managed care may not have serious consequences for physician morale (Baker and Cantor 1993). A more favorable attitude toward managed care seems to be emerging, but many physicians still perceive that managed care has negative consequences for medical practice and physician satisfaction.

Physicians' expectations regarding managed care tend to be more negative than their actual experiences with practice in HMOs (Schulz et al. 1990). This issue was addressed in a community undergoing rapid change in terms of the proportion of the population enrolled in HMOs. In a four-year period, the proportion of the population enrolled in HMOs in Dane County, Wisconsin, increased from 10 percent to over 40 percent. More than eight hundred physicians who were affiliated with the HMOs were surveyed regarding their expectations before and their experiences after this change. Most of these physicians had expected a decline in earnings and in the quality of care, but the majority of them reported that neither declined. These findings suggest that satisfaction levels can be fairly high for physicians in managed care settings.

The current state of the health care environment may make physicians more receptive to HMOs and to managed care generally. Iglehart (1992b) pointed out that physicians are increasingly frustrated with traditional fee-for-service medical practice and with growing interference from government and third-party agencies.

What many doctors seem most incensed about is the increasing intrusive government and third-party oversight of their clinical practices and the need to comply with an increasing number of forms, procedures, and regulations imposed by private and public third parties on them and on the patients they treat (the "hassle factor"). These requirements have left many physicians feeling besieged, under emotional stress, frustrated by their loss of control, and worried about the future of the profession. (Iglehart 1992b, 963)

Although the general picture is positive, some of our findings suggest that managed care may face some significant problems in the future, particularly in the area of primary care. Primary care physicians are currently the focus of much attention, and the provision of primary care is a national concern. Primary care physicians report increasing dissatisfaction and frustration with their roles and practice conditions in all types of settings, and the number of medical students planning to specialize in general medicine, family practice, and other primary care specialties is also declining (Colwill 1992). Many primary care physicians are uncomfortable as "gatekeepers," but they are increasingly expected to serve this function, particularly in HMOs, PPOs, and other managed care systems. As Katz pointed out:

> In some ways, they [primary care physicians] are being asked to "solve" societal problems, social and financial. They are expected to be humane, attentive, continuous caregivers attuned to the biopsychosocial needs of their patients and, at the same time, to be financial "gatekeepers," either through restrictive insurance mechanisms or through the conservative and appropriate use of resources. They are called upon to implement preventive and other clinical guidelines. The list goes on and on. And, despite these responsibilities, they are the least well compensated physicians among all others. (Katz 1992, 4)

Our results showed that primary care physicians were more satisfied than other specialists with their income and benefits but less satisfied than other specialists with many other aspects of practice. Primary care physicians tend to be the most pressured in terms of work load, and this is reflected in their dissatisfaction with control over their schedules and with the time they have available for patients. Control over the pace and routines of work and restrictions on referrals were also concerns for many of the primary care physicians.

Continuing and prolonged dissatisfaction may result in burnout, difficulties with patients, and deterioration in physician performance (Mawardi 1979; Linn et al. 1985; Schmoldt 1991). Some studies suggest that physicians who are more dissatisfied tend to use more tests and procedures and make more referrals (Freeborn, Johnson, and Mullooly 1984; Eisenberg 1986). Dissatisfied physicians are also more likely to engage in inappropriate prescribing patterns, to have more difficulty getting patients to follow the physician's instructions regarding prescribed medications and follow-up appointments, and to have patients with lower levels of satisfaction (Eisenberg 1979; Melville 1980; Eisenberg 1985). Generally, they are less likely to relate well to patients or to inspire a sense of trust among their patients (Mechanic 1975). Thus, both quality of care and efficiency may suffer when there are high levels of physician dissatisfaction among primary care physicians.

The response by some HMOs to problems in primary care is to add more physicians or to give physicians more time for other activities, such as administration, teaching, and research (which results in fewer hours available to see patients). This comes with a price. Either the remaining physicians have to increase their productivity, or more physicians are required. Additional physicians increase the total costs of care and require higher premiums. Increased costs erode HMOs' competitive advantage and are likely to make recruitment of members more difficult. Fundamental problems—such as the need to increase productivity and the need for more effective organization and planning—may not get addressed. The supply of primary care physicians is crucial to the HMO model of practice, and most managed care plans are well aware that a crisis exists in primary care (Katz 1992). A number of innovations aimed at improving primary care are being tried. We discuss several of the most promising of these in our last chapter.

In conclusion, HMO plans should give ongoing attention to enhancing their physicians' work environment and to improving satisfaction among physicians. HMOs are complex systems that require a great deal from physicians in terms of shared commitment, conceptual understanding, and patient care responsibilities. In many ways, our findings are variations on themes echoed over the years in past studies and reviews. In 1969, Avedis Donabedian concluded his review of the performance of prepaid group practice with the following statement:

> The great majority of subscribers and physicians in prepaid group practice are satisfied by what they have. Nevertheless, there are two problems that have not been fully solved: How to promote the full flowering of the professional spirit, and how to nurture the sensitive personal relationships between professionals and their clients in complex bureaucracies that are governed by impersonal exigencies of their own. These are, of course, problems not only of prepaid group practice but of medical care in all organized settings. They are, moreover, problems that face our society in many spheres . . . and that need to be solved on a much broader front. (Donabedian 1969, 27)

6

The Future of Managed Care

> If we do not learn from history, we shall be
> compelled to relive it. True. But if we do not
> change the future, we shall be compelled to endure
> it. And that could be worse.
> —Alvin Toffler

Soaring health care costs and lack of access to care for millions of Americans have led third-party payers and government policy makers to accelerate their efforts to promote managed care as an alternative to insurance plans based on the fee-for-service system. President Clinton's health reform plan strongly emphasizes managed care, as do most of the legislative proposals to reform the health care system. Business leaders see managed care as the best hope for controlling costs and for preserving private providers' and payers' dominance over the health care system; and many government policy makers see managed care as a way of achieving demonstrable savings in Medicare and Medicaid and expanding coverage to the uninsured. However, the idea of managed care is still new to many Americans, who place great importance on unrestricted choice of physicians and health plans.

Health care reform through universal access to some form of health insurance is highly likely in the foreseeable future. Almost all the proposals for reform maintain some choice of health plans and providers but include incentives for both individuals and providers to affiliate with managed care plans (Enthoven and Kronick 1991). Managed care that integrates the financing, organizing, and delivery of medical services into a single system represents a major departure from traditional health insurance, which has been mainly a mechanism for financing medical care. In this chapter, we focus on this integrated model of managed care, best represented by the prepaid group practice HMO. The other models are basically variations on traditional fee-for-service medical practice and do not in any fundamental sense change the financing of services, the way in which physicians are paid, or the way in which medical practice is organized. Moreover, information on the performance of these plans is too limited to serve as a basis for firm conclusions.

Though the relative cost effectiveness of HMOs is now generally accepted, other aspects of this form of managed care remain major concerns of both policy makers and potential enrollees. In this book we have examined various aspects of this form of managed care to address the question of how its performance measures up to the potential of managed care generally. We now ask: Is it feasible or realistic to expect that this form of managed care can be implemented on a national basis? Will consumers voluntarily join HMOs, accepting constraints on their choice of physicians and on other aspects of care? Can HMOs recruit physicians and provide them with a satisfying work environment? Will physicians accept greater controls over their practice patterns? If this form of managed care can be implemented on a national basis, will it provide access to care for all Americans? Will it contribute to a continuous improvement in the quality of care available in this country?

We address these issues in light of what we have learned from our own research and observations and from the literature regarding managed health care. In this chapter, we go beyond our data and the Kaiser Permanente, Northwest Region, setting to discuss some of the major issues that will need to be addressed as the organization, financing, and delivery of health care continue to evolve in the United States. We conclude by offering several thoughts on the reforming of the U.S. medical care system.

Serving a Diverse Population

Our findings and those of others who have studied populations enrolled in HMOs clearly indicate that HMOs can satisfy the needs of most patients and that, given the choice, a significant proportion of the population will join this type of managed care plan. A key question about the population that enrolls in HMOs has been whether HMOs attract healthier people and practice "skimming." Some biased selection does seem to occur (largely for reasons outside the control of the HMO), but as HMOs mature they also attract and retain people who are less healthy. The longer people continue their membership, the more their health reflects their lifestyles and the aging process, factors essentially unrelated to the original enrollment decision.

Our data for a large, well-established HMO show its members to be highly similar in their sociodemographic characteristics to the community population and to the population enrolled in conventional plans. Selection—or, more accurately, retention—of a particular health insurance plan becomes at some point a matter of habit or inertia. And even with first-time selection among choices, a variety of non-economic and non-health-related factors are paramount. These include acceptance of what is familiar or what is recommended by friends, co-workers, or other trusted persons.

Many policy makers and employers, however, believe that HMOs are cost-effective because they disproportionately attract healthy, low-risk individuals and this selection effect gives them a competitive advantage. Employers have responded by developing strategies that impose different cost-sharing requirements on different classes of employees. More and more employers are moving toward experience rating and greater cost sharing by employees (Hornbrook 1991). This strategy results in an increase in the number of people without health insurance or with inadequate coverage. The people most affected tend to be those who are the sickest and those who are chronically ill or disabled—those who need the most care and are the most vulnerable members of our society.

This situation has led to the need for better risk-adjustment mechanisms to adjust premiums across plans to reflect differences in the risks the plans are assuming through enrollment. Better knowledge of risks would allow managed care plans to develop options for adjusting employer contributions to compensate for selection effects (Hornbrook 1991). Current risk-adjustment methods are very inadequate, however, and this area will have to be addressed if managed care and "managed competition" become national policy.

Managed care is at best a partial solution to the health care crisis if it can serve only the working and middle classes. Any consideration of managed care plans must include an assessment of their capacity to integrate currently underserved groups, such as the poor, into their delivery systems. Of course, the underlying problem of access cannot be fully solved until some form of universal health insurance coverage or financial subsidy exists for those without access to employment-based insurance or adequate personal financial resources. The contribution of managed care is to demonstrate the advantages of a more rational organization of medical care services, rather than to solve the problem of financing the full cost of such services.

A number of demonstrations in the 1960s and early 1970s showed that it is possible to incorporate the poor into HMOs if public financing is available (Greenlick 1971). Evaluations of these programs indicated that for poor people enrolled in HMOs the cost of care was lower, while access to care and the quality of the care provided were as good as or better than they would have been under fee-for-service financing. When the poor had access to primary care physicians and other services, their utilization patterns soon became very similar to that of the general membership (Greenlick et al. 1972). The poor reduced their use of the emergency room and increased their use of regular preventive care (e.g., immunizations and prenatal care) and ongoing primary care. Though there are major problems to be overcome, the evidence suggests that at least the large, mature HMOs can successfully integrate the care of underserved populations into their programs.

Another significant challenge relates to the question of whether managed care can effectively serve the elderly. Medicare members are the fastest-growing segment of KPNW enrollees, for example; and whether HMOs and other forms of managed care can succeed financially while absorbing increasing numbers of older people is still an open question. Some Medicare prospective payment demonstrations in HMOs suggest that older populations can be successfully integrated into managed care settings (Greenlick et al. 1983). However, this issue will be a formidable challenge for managed care.

Rural populations also present a difficult challenge, though integrated delivery systems are working in some rural areas (Kent 1993). However, fully integrating rural areas and populations into managed care systems will require urban-based systems to create rural satellites linked through state-of-the-art communication and transportation systems. Through these linkages primary care providers—physicians, nurse practitioners, and others—can have quick and easy access to medical information and specialists. Some types of specialty care can also be provided in rural settings through a regular schedule of periodic visits from the urban-based system. Of course, tertiary care would be provided only in the urban setting of the managed care system, but the rural satellites would have access to such care via a variety of communication and transportation links. Provision for these integrated rural-urban systems would, of course, have to be built into the financing mechanism; such mechanisms and systems might well be created through existing medical schools and teaching hospitals. Not only would this help fund these increasingly costly enterprises, it could also help in the ongoing reformulation of medical education and training necessary for keeping up with technological change and the health care needs of the American population.

As the U.S. population continues to age, special demands will be placed on the medical care system. Aging, and other social trends in the larger society, will challenge the health care system to develop better ways of dealing with people who have chronic diseases and/or physical and mental disabilities. HMOs offer the opportunity to deal with these challenges in an integrated way. Improving primary care and incorporating long-term care into the continuum of care are challenges that HMOs will need to meet to increase quality while maintaining control over costs. A number of innovations are being tried in this area, but most of these have not been evaluated or widely implemented. Models that emphasize aggressive case management and treatment planning for patients with multiple and complex problems are examples (Kramer, Fox, and Morgenstern 1992).

These new models require the reshaping of patient-physician relationships to involve and empower patients so that they can participate more actively in their own care and in the management of their chronic conditions. These models require physicians to give up some of their autonomy and to work cooperatively with other allied health professionals and team members. This can probably best be achieved inside a system where all stand to benefit by modifying traditional ways of relating to one another. The individualistic, biologically oriented model of care worked reasonably well for acute diseases but is dysfunctional when the major problem is the management of chronic disease and disability (Mechanic 1986).

HMOs provide an advantageous environment in which to test and implement innovations in primary care and new treatment models. In a number of areas, we already have considerable knowledge, but implementation of new approaches has been slow (Katz 1992). HMOs have a greater capacity to develop better ways of managing care for persons with chronic disease and integrating ambulatory care with long-term care than do other currently available options (Greenberg et al. 1988). Many HMOs, for example, have programs in place for particular groups of patients with chronic conditions, but more comprehensive systems need to be developed for the full range of chronically ill patients—those patients needing multiple medical and supportive services, as well as those who have chronic diseases that are asymptomatic but who need careful monitoring and preventive care (Kramer, Fox, and Morgenstern 1992).

HMOs have a great potential for efficiently and more rapidly responding to the expanding knowledge about disease prevention and health promotion. Rates of immunizations, Pap smears, mammography screening, and the like have been found to be higher for HMO members than for others, although the levels are still less than what has been recommended by the U.S. Centers for Disease Control and Prevention, the medical profession, and public health agencies (Greenlick, Freeborn, and Pope 1988). HMOs have rarely developed ongoing systems to ensure high levels of prevention in their populations, but they are moving in that direction. The technology (e.g., computerized registries and administrative and clinical information systems that can be used to identify at-risk individuals) is available to make this economically feasible, so if there are further incentives such systems will be implemented.

Although HMOs can successfully integrate disadvantaged groups into their membership, their total membership still has to be balanced so that the population to be served includes a cross-section of the socioeconomic spectrum. Attempts to develop HMOs that served only or mostly disadvantaged populations were not successful. That is, a number of the early demonstrations failed because they limited their membership to the poor. The plans ultimately could not be sustained because the resulting high utilization and costs could not be supported by the available financing.

Meeting Consumer Needs

The existing evidence demonstrates that staff- and group-model HMO managed care systems have a major effect on use and costs of services for their members, and these results are reflected in members' attitudes. Members in HMO managed care plans have consistently seen reduced costs and broad coverage as major advantages of this form of care. The costs have been lower because these managed care systems have been able to contain utilization rather than because they are more efficient producers of medical care (Luft 1978).

However, managed care places on patients various constraints that could limit consumer acceptability and the widespread growth of managed care. In most managed care systems, members are required to see only physicians who are members of the plan's panel. In addition, patients usually have to choose a primary care physician who controls access to other services. This leads to the fear on the part of some that managed care will restrict access and delay needed treatment. Related to this fear is the concern that the bureaucratic nature of managed care will result in impersonal care. Most of these concerns seem unfounded.

Our data on consumer satisfaction show that most KPNW members are well satisfied with the quality of care they receive and with how they are treated by physicians and other staff members and providers. Although patients feel some constraints on their choice of provider and express dissatisfaction with their access to routine care, they are generally satisfied with most other aspects of care and service. They tend to weigh their dissatisfaction with some aspects of access to care against the advantages of more comprehensive coverage at lower cost, and the availability of a system of care when they "really need it."

Our findings also showed that the views of patients and physicians are congruent regarding the advantages and disadvantages of KPNW for patients. Both groups see price, comprehensive benefits, and the lack of "hassle" regarding forms, paperwork, and the like as major advantages. The availability of a broad range of specialists and the provision of high-quality care are also viewed as significant pluses. The perceptions of the two groups are also congruent regarding the disadvantages of KPNW. Both physicians and patients view access to routine care and continuity of care as problematic, and both express frustration regarding various "bureaucratic" aspects of managed care—such as the difficulty of getting through the system to talk with a physician and of getting a non-emergency appointment.

As Mechanic stated it, consumers are likely to view HMOs and other managed care systems in much the same way as they view large department stores or retail chains:

> The consumer generally understands that he or she gets a reasonable product for a reasonable price. He is unlikely to find the very best, and amenities may be lacking to some degree, but the consumer perceives a relatively good deal for his money. Occasionally, such a well-managed store will provide more amenities than expected, and occasional products may be better than those found at more luxurious establishments, but the usual expectation is a reliable product at a fair price. (Mechanic 1986, 70)

This suggests that if HMOs are to compete successfully in the long run, they will have to do more than change one or two specific aspects of service. To produce high levels of member satisfaction, they must improve services across the system, especially in those areas where members are the least satisfied (e.g., waiting time for routine appointments, time spent on the phone making appointments, time spent waiting to see the physician, the difficulty of seeing one's own physician, interaction with the physician, and the responsiveness of physicians generally). Recent studies suggest that, cumulatively, making improvements in these areas can dramatically increase the number of highly satisfied members (Robertson 1993).

While HMOs, to increase patient satisfaction, must continue to innovate in the organization and delivery of care, the "demand side" of care must also be more appropriately managed. That is, knowledge and information must be made more available to consumers at a level they can understand, so that they can use it to manage their own health—not only by sharing more in the medical decisions affecting them directly, and by assuming more responsibility for their lifestyles and behavior, but also by being able to better determine when care is needed and what level of professional service is required. With better knowledge, people will elect care and treatment in keeping with their personal needs and values, and from the provider qualified to give it, even if this is not a physician, whether a generalist or a specialist. At the same time, having better or more complete knowledge about the benefits and risks of care will change people's expectations of the medical care system. All of this can have a positive effect on the cost and quality of care. Current studies of "shared decision making" are already beginning to demonstrate this (Wennberg 1990).

As many studies have shown, people are not well informed about alternative insurance plans or health care systems and lack even the most basic information about their differential advantages and disadvantages. A national effort to educate people and to provide objective information about alternative plans is sorely needed. Consumers must be better informed if they are to assume responsibility for their health care choices, a concept now being articulated by policy makers and others interested in achieving health care reform. If medical costs are to be contained, and the quality of care maintained or improved, people need to be aware of the consequences of their health care decisions. Mechanic, Ettel, and Davis pointed out that "as managed care becomes a more central aspect of health care in general, it is essential that patients understand how such medical care plans work. Whatever restriction of options takes place in the future, informed choice among the alternatives available is likely to contribute to the quality of patient satisfaction and to minimize disruption in the care process" (Mechanic, Ettel, and Davis 1990, 23).

Improving Ambulatory Care

The future success of managed care systems will also depend on their ability to improve the delivery of ambulatory care and to provide it more efficiently. Although HMOs have reduced inpatient utilization, they have not achieved great efficiency in the delivery of ambulatory care, and many physicians who practice in HMO settings are frustrated with the current ways of organizing and providing ambulatory care. Already some HMOs are trying new approaches for organizing ambulatory care. These include primary care module systems that serve defined panels of patients, and case management for patients with multiple and complex problems.

Module panel systems attempt to make work loads more equitable and encourage physicians and allied health professionals to work together as teams. Continuity of care is emphasized. Each primary care team has a defined group of patients who are the responsibility of the team; and each patient selects a personal physician or allied health professional within the module and is expected to receive care from the provider chosen. But if the patient's primary care provider is not available, the patient will receive care from one of the other clinicians in the module. Patients seeking medical advice have their questions answered by someone working within the module, and the provider team is responsible for health appraisals (i.e., physical examinations) and urgent care. These changes are intended to increase both the quality of primary care and the efficiency of its delivery. These efforts, however, need to be systematically evaluated.

Various triage mechanisms, such as systems in which patients first speak to advice or triage nurses, are also used in some HMO settings, and a number of HMOs use nurse practitioners and physician assistants to provide routine ambulatory care. Few managed care plans make maximal use of these types of personnel, even though they have been found to be effective and to enhance patient satisfaction. More effort needs to be directed toward determining the most effective and efficient combinations of medical personnel for delivering different kinds of medical care services.

Even though we found that KPNW members with poorer health tended to have a regular provider, we also found that many members did not. In fact, a significant proportion of members in our studies said they did not think it especially important to have a personal or regular physician; having a regular source of care seemed to be more important, particularly for healthy people. Still, there are advantages to having a regular physician, regardless of one's age and health status. For example, the quality and continuity of care would likely be better, and patient satisfaction would be enhanced. Patients who are more satisfied are less likely to use services outside the plan or to terminate their membership. Much more could be done by HMOs and other forms of managed care to link people with a regular primary care provider.

Many HMOs have developed policies and procedures to make sure that every new member has the opportunity to choose a regular primary care provider and to make an initial visit. This provides baseline information on the member's health status and provides an opportunity to assist the new member in understanding how best to use the health care system. It may also help to get the physician-patient relationship off to a sound start. Similar procedures can be developed to make sure that every long-time member of a given plan has the opportunity to choose a regular primary care provider and has access to that provider when needed.

It is important to note that measuring the continuity of care is a complex task, and that investigators usually have settled for determining whether a person has a personal physician. A few research studies have used an episode approach to measure the utilization of services and the continuity of care (Luft 1981; Hornbrook and Berki 1985; Hornbrook, Hurtado, and Johnson 1985). With this method, one can track where people go for care and can identify discontinuities and lack of coordination and follow-up. This approach requires complex data systems to measure the services provided and the procedures performed, and to track referrals and consultations, the degree of compliance with medical recommendations, the follow-up of abnormal findings, and treatment outcomes for specific morbidities. Because of the expense and complexity of the episode approach, few HMOs monitor continuity in this way.

In the future, HMOs will be under much greater pressure to show that they can improve access to care and the continuity of care while containing costs. This situation will force them to put in place data systems for monitoring both access and the outcomes of care. As Patrick and Erickson pointed out, policy makers and health care systems will increasingly have to address two fundamental questions: "What is beneficial health care?" and "How should public monies be expended to provide this care to as many people as possible?" (Patrick and Erickson 1993, 338).

Enhancing Physician Performance

Our research and other recent studies show that the HMO setting can provide a satisfying work environment for physicians—at least for those who choose this model of practice. Fears that professional autonomy and the quality of care will suffer have little grounding in reality and are not supported by existing research. Although many community physicians still have concerns about managed care, more are beginning to recognize that it has numerous advantages. Many of the concerns of community physicians about loss of autonomy, reduced incomes, poor quality of care, and the like have been overstated and are not the key problems experienced by physicians in HMOs. The most significant issues have to do with control over the work environment, participation in decisions affecting work life, lack of understanding of and commitment to managed care, and a sense of loss of control.

These problems are expressed in terms of physician dissatisfaction with patient load, time for patients, referral procedures, lack of control over schedule, and lack of ability to affect the work environment. Many physicians also feel that HMOs make it difficult to maintain stability of patient relationships and continuity of care. These dissatisfactions are not universal among HMO physicians and do not appear to have adversely affected the overall quality of care provided, although they certainly have the potential to affect practice patterns, which in turn could affect both the quality and the cost of care.

These concerns are more problematic for primary care physicians, who serve as "gatekeepers" in managed care settings. Although physicians generally support the concept of gatekeeping, the gatekeeper role is stressful for many primary care physicians. In the immediate future, unless more effective means are found to balance demand and the provision of services, primary care physicians may face increasing conflicts between their role as patient advocate—which may involve striving to do everything conceivably possible, and then some, for patients—and their resource allocation role, which seeks to balance the use of resources against the value of the outcome (Mechanic 1986). The fact that older primary care physicians tend to be much more satisfied with this role may suggest that, as physicians learn the new role, they may find it less stressful and learn to accept it more easily.

In the future, managed care systems must be able to attract and retain large numbers of qualified primary care practitioners. Recruitment of primary care physicians, however, is a growing national problem, and the lack of primary care physicians could become a limiting factor for the growth of managed care. Competition for physicians among managed care organizations and other systems is likely to increase significantly, particularly if current trends in specialty choice continue. The future success of HMOs will depend in large part on their ability to improve the efficiency of ambulatory care and to improve satisfaction levels for primary care physicians (Katz 1992). To some degree, these are competing goals and present HMOs with complex and challenging problems: can HMOs find ways both to be more efficient in the delivery of ambulatory care and to improve quality and provider satisfaction?

We should note that trends in medical education affect physician recruitment and physicians' attitudes about practicing in managed care plans. As Luft (1981) pointed out, much of primary care physicians' dissatisfaction with patient care may result from inappropriate emphasis in medical education, not from HMO policies. Traditionally, the emphasis has been on acute care and hospital-based specialty training. If medical schools continue their emphasis on the training of specialist rather than generalist physicians, managed care organizations may encounter ongoing problems in providing primary care. Considerable pressures exist to increase the supply of generalists and to restructure medical education to take account of the needs of society and new forms of practice (Greenlick 1992; Katz 1992). Reforms in medical education, however, are difficult to achieve, and fundamental change is unlikely in the immediate future. In the meantime, managed care systems will have to address the very real problems in primary care and continue to seek ways to organize it more efficiently. As the population ages, this issue becomes even more problematic.

A key characteristic of successful managed care systems is effective working relationships between physicians and nonphysician managers. The most successful systems have missions, cultures, and policies that integrate physicians into all aspects of management and governance activities (Shortell 1991). Many managed care plans tend to emphasize efficiency and instrumental activities but neglect the integrative activities that are so important for sustaining motivation and commitment to the organization as a whole (Etzioni 1965; Greenlick 1989).

As managed care systems increase in size and complexity, decision making becomes more centralized, and bureaucratic control mechanisms are instituted to improve productivity and quality. This can increase levels of both physician and patient dissatisfaction. Avoiding these problems may require changes in administrative structures to allow more participation by physicians in decision making on issues that affect the work environment and their day-to-day work life. Increasing physicians' opportunities to participate in management and in policy decisions has been shown to improve satisfaction and organizational commitment as well as quality of care (Barr and Steinberg 1983; Shortell 1991). More formally planned mechanisms to orient new physicians to the conditions of practice and to socialize them to the values and norms of practice in managed care settings are also necessary.

In recruiting physicians, however, expectations should not be raised beyond what is achievable. Physicians should be given realistic information about what to expect regarding work load, casemix, and the demands of practice (Schulz et al. 1990). There is a growing management literature on how to involve physicians in organizational life and how to improve relationships with physicians (Shortell and Kaluzny 1988; Shortell 1991). Probably nothing is more important to the successful operation of a managed care system than a medical staff that works in harmony with the organization. This requires the development of a shared organizational culture that respects physician autonomy and professional goals while recognizing the legitimate domains of management. Creating this culture requires both the physicians and the managers to be committed to the goals of managed care—the provision of efficiently organized, high-quality medical care that is both affordable and satisfying to the population it serves.

Outcomes research and practice guidelines are strategies that are being promoted nationally to improve the quality of medical care and to make treatment more efficient. Physicians vary widely in the way they practice, and implementation of these strategies could reduce variation in physician practice patterns and reduce costs (Eisenberg 1986; Berwick 1991). The development of outcomes research (to determine what works and what doesn't work) and practice guidelines research is based on the assumption that dissemination of guidelines will eliminate inefficient and ineffective practices in both fee-for-service and managed care settings. The development of practice guidelines and better outcomes data systems is certainly a step in the right direction and should be strongly supported. These innovations are significant for managed care because their application in practice could help to ensure that resources are allocated on the basis of medical need and not patients' social characteristics or the pressures of practice. In general, physicians favor the development of practice guidelines and outcomes research. But they will have to be convinced that they can control the process of implementation of the practice guidelines (Berwick 1991). So far, we do not know if physicians will adapt their practice to guidelines, and little conclusive evidence exists on whether guidelines affect the costs and quality of medical care (Brook 1989). Some critics maintain that practice guidelines will lead to "cookbook medicine" and may be used as an excuse to limit services when people really need them.

Before practice guidelines are widely implemented, outcomes research should be expanded to determine what processes are most successful in implementing guidelines in different settings, and the effects of guidelines in alternative systems of care. It may be naive to expect that their implementation can succeed without changes in fee-for-service reimbursement or other structural factors that play an important role in physician behavior.

Other approaches for changing physician behavior, such as continuous quality improvement (CQI) and confidential feedback on physicians' use of lab tests and x rays, and on prescribing patterns and the like, may also be useful for reducing costly variation in practice patterns. Many physicians, however, are skeptical and feel that these are management gimmicks to control physicians' decision making and to limit professional autonomy (Berwick 1991). At present, evidence is lacking on the cost effectiveness of these approaches and on the feasibility of implementing practice guidelines on a wide scale. If these techniques are imposed without physicians' input and ongoing participation, they will surely fail.

Too often, managers have proposed technocratic solutions to what in reality are social and political problems. Fundamental issues and genuine differences about who should control medical work and the allocation of resources are often ignored. To be successful, techniques such as CQI and practice guidelines will have to be shown to improve outcomes and the quality of physicians' work life. The assumptions underlying these types of changes should be examined in light of their psychosocial effects on both patients and physicians and on the extent to which they are likely to achieve more humane and productive ways of organizing medical work (Karasek 1979; Karasek and Theorell 1990).

Increasing Prevention and Health Promotion

Most HMOs have done very little in the areas of health promotion and disease prevention (Vogt 1993). Costs, lukewarm support by physicians and managers, high member turnover, and other factors have been cited as reasons for neglecting this area (Luft and Morrison 1991). Also cited is the lack of knowledge about what really works to change behavior in health-enhancing ways.

Much more could be done by existing HMOs to improve health levels in the populations they serve. For example, they could establish yearly population-based preventive targets (e.g., to reduce smoking levels, to increase the use of seat belts, and/or to decrease the percentage of low-birth weight infants) and design and evaluate programs targeted to achieve these objectives.

Programs of prevention and health maintenance could also be designed for middle-aged and older adults to maintain or increase their functional health status and perhaps lower their overall use of services, and the associated costs. A major deterrent to this kind of effort is the lack of data systems to measure health status and to monitor changes in health status over time. Few managed care settings have the capacity to provide this kind of data, and we currently have no national data system with which to compare different health plans on these kinds of things. This is a national issue and one that must be addressed if we are ever going to be able to compare the performance of different approaches to the financing and provision of health care services.

Future Policy Issues

Over the past decade, hybrid plans—for instance, IPAs, PPOs, and point-of-service plans—have developed that combine features of managed care with features of traditional indemnity insurance. These new plans represent strategies not only to meet the demands of employers for better control over their health care costs through greater variability in benefits and more cost sharing with employees than HMO plans generally allow, but also to meet the demands of consumers for more freedom to choose providers than HMO plans provide. However, the blurred distinction between traditional indemnity plans and managed care makes it difficult to compare their performance and understand what it is about them that would explain any differences in their performance (Luft and Morrison 1991). There is a need for a better conceptual framework for distinguishing among the essential elements of the various plans so that they can be meaningfully classified and compared as to their performance across a number of different dimensions (Hornbrook and Berki 1985). Hornbrook and Goodman (1991), for example, propose a classification system based on differentiations among the following elements: restrictions on patient choice, restrictions on physician autonomy, risk-based payment, and vertical integration. Until we have a meaningful classification system, we will have little potential for comparing the performance of the more recent hybrid managed care plans with that of HMO–managed care plans.

Although many key policy makers strongly support managed care and "managed competition," the population at large is concerned that their individual preferences and needs, and the freedom of physicians to make clinical judgments, will be compromised by managed care. The fear is that quality and access will be sacrificed for cost controls. The need for public accountability to ensure that access and quality are not compromised can be met through ongoing evaluation and monitoring of the performance of alternative health care systems. This will require the collection and reporting of uniform data, including data that represents the views and experience of members. There is now sufficient evidence that measures based on member reports can be highly reliable (or reproducible) and accurate (or valid) indicators of various aspects of medical care delivery and treatment. Currently, we have no uniform data systems to measure the performance of alternative health care systems. But many employers and third-party agencies are now asking managed care plans to provide this kind of information. We can expect government also to require this information if managed care becomes part of the proposed solution to the health care crisis in the United States.

A significant advantage of staff- and group-model HMOs is their ability to develop a database reflecting the utilization experience of a defined and known population, and to examine that utilization in light of the demographic characteristics of the population. This ability provides the foundation for further research on the performance of managed care. This point is often unrecognized, or unappreciated, by managers and policy makers, but any viable national system of accountability for managed care must be population-based. Without this capability, making meaningful comparisons among alternative plans will be very difficult.

With health care reform there is an opportunity for medical care in the United States to become population-based—that is, focused on improving or maintaining the health of a defined population rather than simply providing services to individual patients who come into the provider's office, the emergency room, or the hospital. A managed care system has the potential for proactively organizing the delivery of care so as to achieve predetermined goals relating to prevention (e.g., immunization of children), detection and early intervention (e.g., screening of populations at risk), and treatment (e.g., treatment of patients with chronic conditions such as asthma and diabetes). A managed care system can also find ways to work collaboratively with the population for which it is accountable, in order to define health care needs and determine how best to go about meeting them. In short, the system can focus on the population and its needs while the individual provider can continue to deliver care to individual patients.

Presently, managed care plans do not have the data systems in place to respond to the requests or demands of business or government. To meet this challenge, however, the managed care industry has proposed the development of a performance measurement system to be used nationwide to compare the quality of care and other dimensions of performance of managed care systems (Priest 1993). Not determined yet is who will participate in this effort, how it will be funded, how the performance measures will be developed, and how the data will be collected. The basic purpose is to develop a common data set and a performance measurement system that will assist managed care plans in improving the quality of care provided to their members and that will allow consumers and purchasers to make more informed choices in their selection of plans.

To be successfully implemented, such a measurement system will have to overcome formidable technical and organizational problems and will require large amounts of funding. Developing the kind of systems required is a complex task and will probably take a number of years. However, health care reform, and governmental requirements for accountability, could speed up the development of a national uniform data set for measuring performance. Not only could such a data system serve to monitor health care delivery in the United States, but it could also contribute to the development and testing of innovations to improve the organization and delivery of health care services.

Realizing the Promise—Some Final Thoughts

Rising costs continue to be the central issue in health care, and the growth of managed care has not stemmed the ever rising tide of national health care expenditures (Rice 1992). Medical costs have continued to rise at a rate much greater than that of inflation in the general economy. Managed care plans are still relatively new, and much of the U.S. population remains covered by conventional insurance plans, which reimburse physicians on a fee-for-service basis. Most Medicare and Medicaid recipients also continue to receive services through fee-for-service arrangements. Few observers expect that managed care alone will solve the cost problem. This will depend on other fundamental structural changes (Iglehart 1992a).

As is now well known, a growing number of Americans have no real access to comprehensive medical care. Without universal coverage, disadvantaged groups—persons with low incomes, the unemployed, and many sick or disabled people—will continue to face access problems and to receive fragmented and poor-quality care. President Clinton has placed reform of the health care system at the top of the national agenda. However, given current political realities, radical or fundamental changes seem unlikely. But given also that the current rate of spending on medical care cannot be sustained, further changes in the health care system are inevitable.

In our view, the organization and administration of health care must be carried out through publicly accountable mechanisms to ensure responsiveness to public needs. Federal, state, and local government health agencies should have a major role in planning and evaluating health services, as should consumers and providers.

Americans' belief in the right of all to health care is bringing about major changes in the institutional structure of our society. It is our hope that as a society we will meet the challenge of that belief by creating systems that truly humanize the treatment of people's diseases and promote the health of "all the people." To accomplish this, we might do well, this time around, to heed the advice that one member of the Committee on the Costs of Medical Care offered more than half a century ago:

> The turbulent stream of change which hurries us towards an unknown future is not going to be stayed while we cautiously tinker and solemnly debate the next step. The plain truth is that, rich as the country is in potential wealth, the haphazard system of private medical enterprise is a luxury we cannot afford. ... Only a venture which promises the conservation of "the common health" ... is worthy of the values which are the stakes. If we are to have what may be ours, we must be wise and bold. (CCMC 1972, 199–200)

Data Sources, Survey Design and Analysis, and Multivariate Tables

Data Sources

The data presented in this book have come from a variety of sources. We have briefly described most of these in the text, and for each of the figures and tables we have cited the source of the data. The major sources have been the membership information processing system maintained by Kaiser Permanente, Northwest Region, for administrative purposes, and information systems that the Center for Health Research has designed or helped to create for research purposes. These latter include surveys conducted since the mid-1970s of the KPNW membership and of the Northwest Permanente physicians. Some, but not all, of the questions in the surveys have remained the same across time.

For much of our analysis and presentation we have used data from the 1985 Current Membership Survey. We have done this for several reasons. A primary reason is that the 1985 survey population comprised the sample for the Outpatient Utilization System (described below), and thus we could link data from the survey with information from the outpatient medical records of subscribers and other members of their subscriber units (families). Other reasons were that most of the questions pertinent to this book were asked in the 1985 membership survey, and that by determining which of the 1985 subscriber units were still enrolled five years later (in 1990) and which were not (for reasons other than death, of course) we could address the issue of health plan termination and confirm or update findings from the termination studies we conducted during the 1970s. Other than this, and for other data sources, we have used the most recent data available. Because our various studies and analyses over the years have shown results that are highly consistent with what we report in this book, we think that our generalizations are valid.

KPNW Administrative Databases

THE MEMBERSHIP INFORMATION PROCESSING SYSTEM

KPNW maintains a Membership Information Processing System (MIPS) to identify past and present KPNW members and to serve the organization's administrative and financial needs. MIPS maintains the base of membership data and employer group data to support member identification, group contract and benefit administration, group and direct-pay billing, and membership and revenue reporting. MIPS is an on-line update, inquiry, and batch reporting system. MIPS data are transferred to a relational database with two major components— current eligibility for care, which has information on all persons who are currently eligible or who terminated within the past year, and historical eligibility, which has information on all persons who have ever been members of KPNW.

THE KAISER APPOINTMENT/REGISTRATION/ ENCOUNTER SYSTEM

The Kaiser Appointment/Registration/Encounter System (KARE) was established in 1985 and provides data on medical office visits for each KPNW member. The primary purpose of this administrative system is to assist medical offices in managing appointments. The KARE system provides the sampling frame for the selection of visits included in the Surveys of Medical Office Visits conducted since 1991 by the Center for Health Research. Comparisons of the appointment lag times determined by using 1992 data from the KARE system with the lag times reported in the 1992 patient office visit survey showed highly similar patterns, thus supporting the use of patient reports as valid and reliable indicators of accessibility.

Center for Health Research Databases

THE OUTPATIENT UTILIZATION SYSTEM

Since 1966, the CHR has maintained an outpatient utilization database (the Outpatient Utilization System, or OPUS) for a continuously updated sample of the KPNW membership. Each month, a simple random sample (a 5% sample from 1966 through 1986; a 2% sample since 1987) of all new KPNW subscriber units is added to the pool of members whose records are then abstracted ever afterwards. All symptoms and all morbidities are recorded for each visit. A morbidity coding system, the KPNW Disease Classification System, was designed for OPUS when the system began in 1966 and has been continuously expanded since that time. This system was originally adapted from *International Classification of Diseases* (USDHEW 1962). Through table look-up procedures the morbidity coding can be grouped according to other disease classification systems. Physicians and other medical care providers serve as consultants to the abstracters, both routinely and when questions arise that require special clarification. The abstracting unit is staffed by accredited record technicians or equivalent personnel. A full year of apprenticeship is required for complete training in this system.

KPNW subscribers in the OPUS sample who participated in the 1985 Current Membership Survey (see below) comprise the basic study population for chapter 3 ("Access and Continuity in Managed Care"). To control for differences in eligibility for care, we further limited the sample to the 80 percent of this population who were in KPNW for the two full years 1985–86. This sample represents the largest and most stable component of the KPNW population. Its patterns of utilization (as a population) tend to be highly consistent from year to year. Finally, we linked the 1985 Current Membership Survey data with the computerized OPUS data for this population.

THE CURRENT MEMBERSHIP SURVEY SERIES

The CHR has conducted surveys of KPNW subscribers since 1974. The focus of the surveys is satisfaction/dissatisfaction with the KPNW medical care program, but the surveys also obtain other information about KPNW subscribers and their families. These include social and demographic characteristics not included in the KPNW administrative database, and information relating to the health status and health-related behaviors of the subscribers and their families.

A random sample (a 5% sample through 1991 and a 2% sample beginning in 1992) of KPNW subscriber units is surveyed by mail each year (following a procedure that allows for sending out approximately one-twelfth of the questionnaires each month). Response rates are generally in the mid-60-percent range; underrepresented are young subscribers, who tend to be in good health, to use few services, and to terminate their membership for reasons relating to job changes and leaving the geographic area. To our knowledge, this survey series represents one of the longest, if not the longest, continuous data series in the United States about the performance of a medical care program from the perspective of the subscriber. These surveys, especially the 1985 survey, provide most of the data for chapter 4 ("Patient Satisfaction with Managed Care").

THE 1970–1971 HOUSEHOLD INTERVIEW SURVEY

A household interview survey of a sample of KPNW subscriber units (families) was conducted in 1970–71 to obtain extensive social, economic, demographic, attitudinal, health-related, and other data for longitudinal studies. The survey obtained information on all of the nearly 4,400 members of the 1,529 subscriber units that participated in the study (representing a 92% completion rate). Answers to extensive open-ended questions asking members about their satisfaction and dissatisfaction with the KPNW medical care program, and their reasons for joining KPNW, were used in designing the annual membership surveys discussed above. Studies using data from this survey have also contributed to our knowledge of KPNW and of the utilization of medical care services.

THE 1984–1985 COMMUNITY SURVEY

The 1984–85 community household interview survey was designed by the CHR but conducted by a commercial survey research organization to avoid bias through identification with KPNW. The survey used a multistage area probability sample design with replacement to achieve a sample of 1,000 households. Interviews were completed with 997 households in the major geographic areas served by the Northwest Region of Kaiser Permanente—the urbanized areas of Portland and Salem, Oregon, and Vancouver, Washington. The survey included the uninsured as well as the insured. In each of these households, a personal interview using a structured questionnaire (with both fixed-alternative and open-ended questions) was conducted—either with the primary occupant of the household or, if the household contained a married pair, with either of the spouses, who then provided information about the other spouse and the family as a whole. In addition to obtaining basic social and demographic information, and other background information, on the individuals and families surveyed, the survey also obtained information about health insurance coverage (including reasons for selecting whatever plan/plans they were enrolled in), health status, and the use of medical care services. The survey also obtained information about the consumer attitudes and behaviors of those surveyed. This 1984–85 community survey is a basic data source for chapter 2 ("Choosing a Managed Care Plan"). In our analyses we have generally excluded those households headed by a person aged sixty-five or older.

Most of these households were made up of retired people who lived only with a spouse, or alone, and were covered by Medicare.

SURVEYS OF MEDICAL OFFICE VISITS

Since 1991, the CHR has selected a stratified (by facility) random sample of visits to KPNW clinicians for a post-visit survey. Members making the visits are asked a series of questions about the visit, including why they had made the visit, how satisfied/dissatisfied they had been with various components of the visit (e.g., wait times and appointment lags), and how they evaluated the quality of the service and the medical care received. These surveys provide some of the data used in chapter 4 ("Patient Satisfaction with Managed Care"). Although satisfaction/dissatisfaction is inherently subjective, there is research literature to support the use of patient ratings as reliable and valid measures of many aspects of medical care, including the accessibility and quality of care and service (e.g., see Ware, Davies, and Rubin 1988).

SURVEYS OF NWP PHYSICIANS

In 1977, the CHR undertook a survey of physician members of North-west Permanente. The survey included sections on (1) professional background and experience, (2) reasons for joining the HMO, (3) views on work load, patients, and colleagues, (4) attitudes toward KPNW, satisfaction with various aspects of practice in this setting, and career satisfaction (5) attitudes about therapeutics and about professional aspects of care such as quality of care, professional autonomy and freedom, and colleague relations and referrals, (6) views regarding the management structure and how the group is governed, and (7) attitudes about health policy issues such as national health insurance and the advantages and disadvantages of various health plans.

The survey instrument was a self-administered questionnaire mailed to each physician. Before it was implemented in the Northwest Region, it was extensively pretested in other KP sites. The response rate was 70 percent in 1977, when NWP included 178 physicians. The physician survey was conducted again in 1984, with a response rate of 81 percent. By then, the group had grown to 247 physicians. The 1984 questionnaire was similar to the 1977 questionnaire on most items but included a special section on stress and physician burnout. The most recent physician survey was undertaken in 1991, and builds on the past two surveys. Many of the original questions have been retained, but several new sections have been added reflecting new concerns and issues such as practice guidelines, malpractice, AIDS, national health insurance, and the like. By 1991, the medical group comprised 525 physicians. The response rate of the 1991 physician survey was 84 percent.

In the 1977 and 1984 surveys, no significant differences were found between respondents and the profile of all NWP physicians with respect to gender and medical specialty. The respondents, however, tended to be somewhat younger and also had shorter tenure in comparison with the total medical group. The survey respondents and the total medical group tended to be quite similar on basic background characteristics in 1991. The respondents and the total medical group were similar in age, gender, years with NWP, and specialty.

Survey Design and Analysis

The CHR standards for questionnaire design, data collection, coding, and processing are the same as those of high-quality academic survey research organizations. Samples are selected on the basis of scientific sampling theory, and data are analyzed using standard statistical techniques. Though we do not routinely report in the text the statistics by which we evaluated the data, we have attempted to reflect these in the way in which we communicate our findings. Moreover, as a sort of summing up of the findings, we offer in the text (figs. 2.12, 3.7–10, 4.9, and 5.12) simplified presentations of results from our several multivariate analyses (the fuller results of which are given in tables A.1–4).

Our approach to the analysis is generally as follows: we first examine frequency distributions, then we use chi square and correlational techniques (or measures of association) to examine bivariate relationships, and finally, we examine the relationships among a larger set of variables using multivariate techniques. These techniques differ according to the dependent variable and may include multiple discriminant function analysis, logistic regression analysis, and multiple regression. Because multiple regression is probably familiar to more people, and the conclusions are the same regardless of which technique is used, we have presented in this book only the results from multiple regression analysis. For comparing mean values (e.g., for utilization measures such as number of physician office visits), we have used analysis of variance.

Table A.1. Predictors of KPNW Health Plan Choice (Stepwise Regression)

Independent Variables	Health Plan Choice (KP)		
	R^2	R^2 Change	Beta
Cost/coverage (reason for joining)	.123	.123	.334*
Occupation (blue collar)	.156	.033	−.152*
Shopping pattern (mass market)	.177	.021	.147*

Source: Data from CHR 1984–85 Community Survey.

Note: Variables that did not enter the model include education, income, social class, self-reported health status, utilization (visits), and knowledge about health plans.

*$p < .01$

Table A.2. Predictors of KPNW Subscribers' Access to Ambulatory Care (Multiple Regression)

Independent Variables	Betas for Various Types of Care			
	Preventive Care	Acute Care	Chronic Care	Total
Predisposing factors				
Age	.201*	−.001	.172*	.143*
Sex (female)	.237*	.093*	.056	.138*
Marital status (married)	.124*	.017	−.023	−.025
Family size	−.056	.016	−.019	−.009
Education	.085*	.079*	.091	.100*
Social class (higher)	.008	−.042	.043	−.015
Enabling factors				
Income (higher)	−.051	−.027	−.048	−.057
Regular physician (yes)	.102*	.145*	.179*	.214*
Need				
Self-reported health status	.017	−.073*	−.183*	−.188*
	$R^2 = .133$	$R^2 = .048$	$R^2 = .161$	$R^2 = .196$
	$F = 16.75*$	$F = 20.63*$	$F = 20.68*$	$F = 26.02*$

Source: Data from CHR 1985 Current Membership Survey and OPUS.

*$p < .05$

Table A.3. Predictors of Subscribers' Overall Satisfaction with KPNW (Stepwise Regression)

	Overall Satisfaction		
Independent Variables	R^2	R^2 Change	Beta
Satisfaction			
Overall access	.378	.378	.360*
Personal interest of physician	.508	.130	.297*
Cost/premiums	.531	.023	.152*
Technical competence of physician	.543	.012	.151*
Education	.549	.006	-.060*
Age	.552	.003	.068*
Self-reported health status	.553	.001	.038*
Income	.554	.001	-.032*

Source: Data from CHR 1985 Current Membership Survey.

Note: Variables that did not enter the model include social class, sex, visits in last twelve months, and knowledgeable about KP benefits.

* $p < .05$

Table A.4. Predictors of Overall Satisfaction with KPNW among NWP Physicians (Stepwise Regression)

	Satisfaction		
Independent Variables	R^2	R^2 Change	Beta
Satisfaction			
Participation in decision making	.172	.172	.219*
Income	.238	.066	.202*
Schedule control	.268	.029	.179*
Referrals	.283	.015	.144*
Specialty (primary care)	.298	.015	-.150*
Autonomy	.310	.012	.127*

Source: Data from CHR 1991 Survey of NWP Physicians.

Note: Variables that did not enter the model include age, gender, and workload.

* $p < .01$

References

Acito, F. 1978. Consumer decision making and health maintenance organizations: A review. *Medical Care* 16:1–13.

Aday, L. A., and R. Andersen. 1974. A framework for the study of access to medical care. *Health Services Research* 9:208–20.

Aday, L. A., C. E. Begley, D. R. Lairson, and C. H. Slater. 1993. *Evaluating the Medical Care System: Effectiveness, Efficiency, and Equity.* Ann Arbor: Health Administration Press.

Aharony, L., and S. Strasser. 1993. Patient satisfaction: What we know about and what we still need to explore. *Medical Care Review* 50:49–78.

Andersen, R. M., J. Kravits, and O. W. Anderson. 1971. The public's view of the crisis in medical care: An impetus for changing delivery systems? *Economic and Business Bulletin* 24:44–52.

Andersen, R. M., A. McCutcheon, L. A. Aday, G. Y. Chiu, and R. Bell. 1983. Exploring dimensions of access to medical care. *Health Services Research* 18:49–74.

Anderson, O. W., T. Herold, B. Butler, C. Kohrman, and E. Morrison. 1985. *HMO Development: Patterns and Prospects.* Chicago: Pluribus Press.

Ashcraft, M., R. Penchansky, S. E. Berki, R. S. Fortus, and J. Gray. 1978. Expectations and experience of HMO enrollees after one year: An analysis of satisfaction, utilization, and costs. *Medical Care* 16:14–32.

Astrachan, J. H., and B. M. Astrachan. 1989. Medical practice in organized settings: Redefining medical autonomy. *Archives of Internal Medicine* 149:1509–13.

Baker, L. C., and J. C. Cantor. 1993. Physician satisfaction under managed care. *Health Affairs* 12 (suppl.): 258–70.

Banta, H. D. 1990a. Technology assessment in health care. In *Health Care Delivery in the United States,* edited by A. R. Kovner, pp. 381–400. 4th ed. New York: Springer Publishing Co.

———. 1990b. What is health care? In Kovner, ed., *Health Care Delivery in the United States,* pp. 8–30. *See* Banta 1990a.

Barr, J. K. 1983. Physicians' views of patients in prepaid group practice: Reasons for visits to HMOs. *Journal of Health and Social Behavior* 24:244–55.

Barr, J. K., and M. M. Steinberg. 1983. Professional participation in organizational decision making: Physicians in HMOs. *Journal of Community Health* 8:160–73.

Bashshur, R. L., and C. A. Metzner. 1967. Patterns of social differentiation between Community Health Association and Blue Cross–Blue Shield. *Inquiry* 4:23–44.

———. 1970. Vulnerability to risk and awareness of dual choice of health insurance plans. *Health Services Research* 5:106–13.

Bashshur, R. L., C. A. Metzner, and C. Worden. 1967. Consumer satisfaction with group practice: The CHA case. *American Journal of Public Health* 57:1991–99.

Bell, C. W., B. E. Lewis, and M. O. Zelley. 1990. Managed care: Update and future directions. *Journal of Ambulatory Care Management* 13:15–26.

Ben-David, J. 1958. The professional role of the physician in bureaucratized medicine: A study in role conflict. *Human Relations* 11:255–74.

Benjamini, Y., and Y. Benjamini. 1986. The choice among medical insurance plans. *American Economic Review* 76:221–27.

Berenson, R. A. 1991. A physician's view of managed care. *Health Affairs* 10:106–19.

Berki, S. E., and M. L. Ashcraft. 1979. On the analysis of ambulatory utilization: An investigation of the roles of need, access, and price as predictors of illness and preventive visits. *Medical Care* 17:1163–81.

———. 1980. HMO enrollment: Who joins what and why. A review of the literature. *Milbank Memorial Fund Quarterly / Health and Society* 58:588–632.

Berki, S. E., M. Ashcraft, R. Penchansky, and R. S. Fortus. 1977a. Enrollment choice in a multi-HMO setting: The roles of health risk, financial vulnerability, and access to care. *Medical Care* 15:95–114.

———. 1977b. Health concern, HMO enrollment, and preventive care use. *Journal of Community Health* 3:3–31.

Berki, S. E., R. Penchansky, R. S. Fortus, and M. L. Ashcraft. 1978. Enrollment choices in different types of HMOs: A multivariate analysis. *Medical Care* 16:682–97.

Berwick, D. M. 1991. Practice guidelines: Promise or threat? *HMO Practice* 5:174–77.

Bice, T. W. 1975. Risk vulnerability and enrollment in a prepaid group practice. *Medical Care* 13:698–703.

Bice, T. W., R. L. Eichhorn, and P. D. Fox. 1972. Socioeconomic status and use of physician services: A reconsideration. *Medical Care* 10:261–71.

Bice, T. W., D. L. Rabin, B. H. Starfield, and K. L. White. 1973. Economic class and use of physician services. *Medical Care* 11:287–96.

Bittker, T. E. 1984. Physician expectations and the changing culture of medical practice: Can we adapt? *Group Health Journal* 5:2–5.

Black, J. S., and W. Kapoor. 1990. Health promotion and disease prevention in older people: Our current state of ignorance. *Journal of the American Geriatrics Society* 38:168–72.

Blendon, R. J. 1989. Three systems: A comparative survey. *Health Management Quarterly* 11:2–10.

Boxerman, S. B., V. D. Hennelly, and R. S. Woodward. 1984. Analyzing HMO membership patterns: A microcomputer application. *Journal of Ambulatory Care Management* 7:68–78.

Breslau, N., A. H. Novack, and G. Wolf. 1978. Work settings and job satisfaction: A study of primary care physicians and paramedical personnel. *Medical Care* 16:850–62.

Brook, R. H. 1973. Critical issues in the assessment of quality of care and their relationship to HMOs. *Journal of Medical Education* 48 (suppl.): 114–34.

———. 1989. Practice guidelines and practicing medicine. *JAMA* 262:3027–30.

Brown, L. D. 1983. *Politics and Health Care Organization: HMOs as Federal Policy.* Washington, D.C.: Brookings Institution.

Buchanan, J. L., and S. Cretin. 1986. Risk selection of families electing HMO membership. *Medical Care* 24:39–51.

Budenstein, M. J., and V. D. Hennelly. 1980. Deterrents to family enrollment in a prepaid group practice. *Medical Care* 18:649–56.

Budrys, G. 1993. Coping with change: Physicians in prepaid practice. *Sociology of Health and Illness* 15:353–73.

Buller, M. K., and D. B. Buller. 1987. Physicians' communication style and patient satisfaction. *Journal of Health and Social Behavior* 28:375–88.

Burns, L. R., R. M. Andersen, and S. M. Shortell. 1990. The effect of hospital control strategies on physician satisfaction and physician-hospital conflict. *Health Services Research* 25:527–60.

Buss, M. L. 1985. Proposed responses to new challenges: HMOs' second decade, 1983–1993. *Group Health Journal* 6:17–21.

Christianson, J. B. 1980. The impact of HMOs: Evidence and research issues. *Journal of Health Politics, Policy, and Law* 5:354–67.

Cleary, P. D., and B. J. McNeil. 1988. Patient satisfaction as an indicator of quality care. *Inquiry* 25:25–36.

Cockerham, W. C. 1992. *Medical Sociology.* 5th ed. Englewood Cliffs, N.J.: Prentice-Hall.

Coe, R. M. 1978. *Sociology of Medicine.* New York: McGraw-Hill Book Co.

Colombotos, J., and C. Kirchner. 1986. *Physicians and Social Change.* New York: Oxford University Press.

Colwill, J. M. 1992. Where have all the primary care applicants gone? *New England Journal of Medicine* 326:387–93.

Committee on the Costs of Medical Care (CCMC). 1972. Reprint. *Medical Care for the American People.* New York: Arno Press. Original edition, Chicago: University of Chicago Press, 1932.

Cunningham, F. C., and J. W. Williamson. 1980. How does the quality of health care in HMOs compare to that in other settings? An analytic literature review, 1958 to 1979. *Group Health Journal* 1:4–25.

Darsky, B. J., N. Sinai, and S. J. Axelrod. 1958. *Comprehensive Medical Services under Voluntary Health Insurance.* Cambridge: Harvard University Press.

Davie, J. S., B. Goldberg, and D. Rowe. 1974. Consumer acceptance of Yale Health Plan. *Journal of the American College Health Association* 22:325–31.

Davies, A. R., and J. E. Ware, Jr. 1988. Involving consumers in quality of care assessment. *Health Affairs* 7:33–48.

Davies, A. R., J. E. Ware, Jr., R. H. Brook, J. R. Peterson, and J. P. Newhouse. 1986. Consumer acceptance of prepaid and fee-for-service medical care: Results from a randomized controlled trial. *Health Services Research* 21:429–52.

Davis, K. 1988. Health care and the nation's economic and social agenda. *Bulletin of the New York Academy of Medicine* 64:5–14.

———. 1991. Inequality and access to health care. *Milbank Quarterly* 69:253–73.

Davis, K., G. F. Anderson, D. Rowland, and E. P. Steinberg. 1990. *Health Care Cost Containment.* Baltimore: Johns Hopkins University Press.

Densen, P. M., N. R. Deardorff, and E. Balamuth. 1958. Longitudinal analyses of four years of experience of a comprehensive medical care plan. *Milbank Memorial Fund Quarterly* 36:5–45.

Devita, A. J., and D. A. Pearson. 1982. HMO marketing: Determining the importance of facility location in consumer choice. *Journal of Ambulatory Care Management* 5:1–13.

DiCarlo, S., and J. Gabel. 1989. Conventional health insurance: A decade later. *Health Care Financing Review* 10:77–89.

Diehr, P., D. P. Martin, R. Leickly, L. Krueger, N. Silberg, and S. Barchet. 1987. Use of ambulatory health care services in a preferred provider organization. *Medical Care* 25:1033–43.

Diehr, P., N. Silberg, D. P. Martin, V. Arlow, and R. Leickly. 1990. Use of a preferred provider plan by employees of the city of Seattle. *Medical Care* 28:1073–88.

Donabedian, A. 1969. An evaluation of prepaid group practice. *Inquiry* 6:3–27.

———. 1985. Twenty years of research on the quality of medical care, 1964–1984. *Evaluation and the Health Professions* 8:243–65.

Dutton, D. B. 1979. Patterns of ambulatory health care in five different delivery systems. *Medical Care* 17:221–43.

Eisenberg, J. M. 1979. Sociologic influences on decision-making by clinicians. *Annals of Internal Medicine* 90:957–64.

———. 1985. Physician utilization: The state of research about physicians' practice patterns. *Medical Care* 23:461–83.

———. 1986. *Doctors' Decisions and the Cost of Medical Care: The Reasons for Doctors' Practice Patterns and Ways to Change Them.* Ann Arbor, Mich.: Health Administration Press.

Engel, G. V. 1969. The effect of bureaucracy on the professional autonomy of the physician. *Journal of Health and Social Behavior* 10:30–41.

Enthoven, A. C. 1981. *Health Plan: The Only Practical Solution to the Soaring Cost of Medical Care.* Reading, Mass.: Addison-Wesley.

———. 1984. The Rand experiment and economical health care. *New England Journal of Medicine* 310:1528–30.

Enthoven, A. C., and R. Kronick. 1991. Universal health insurance through incentives reform. *JAMA* 265:2532–36.

Etzioni, A. 1965. Dual leadership in complex organizations. *American Sociological Review* 30:688–98.

Faltermayer, E. 1992. Let's really cure the health system. *Fortune* 125:46–58.

Feldman, R., M. Finch, and B. Dowd. 1989. The role of health practices in HMO selection bias: A confirmatory study. *Inquiry* 26:381–87.

Findlay, S. 1992. Medicine by the book. *U.S. News and World Report,* July 6.

Fink, R. 1984. What does it mean to be an HMO physician? In *The Life Cycle of the HMO Physician.* Proceedings of the GHAA's Medical Directors Education Conference, edited by L. C. Robinson and R. S. Bingham, pp. 17–29. Washington, D.C.: Group Health Association of America.

Foley, J. 1992. *Sources of Health Insurance and Characteristics of the Uninsured: Analysis of the March 1991 Current Population Survey.* Washington, D.C.: Employee Benefit Research Institute.

Forthofer, R. N., J. H. Glasser, and N. Light. 1979. Life table analysis of membership retention in an HMO. *Journal of Community Health* 5:46–53.

Fox, P. D. 1990. Foreword: Overview of managed care trends. In National Health Lawyers Association, *The Insider's Guide to Managed Care.* Washington, D.C.: National Health Lawyers Association.

Freeborn, D. K. 1985. Physician satisfaction in a prepaid group practice HMO. *Group Health Journal* 6:3–12.

Freeborn, D. K., and M. R. Greenlick. 1973. Evaluation of the performance of ambulatory care systems: Research requirements and opportunities. *Medical Care* 11 (suppl.): 68–75.

Freeborn, D. K., R. E. Johnson, and J. P. Mullooly. 1984. *Physicians' Use of Ambulatory Care Resources in a Prepaid Group Practice HMO.* Final Report for grant no. 18-P-9799319-02, HCFA. Portland, Ore.: Kaiser Permanente Medical Care Program, Health Services Research Center.

Freeborn, D. K., and C. R. Pope. 1981. Client satisfaction in a health maintenance organization: Providers' perceptions compared to clients' reports. *Evaluation and the Health Professions* 4:275–94.

———. 1982. Health status, utilization, and satisfaction among enrollees in three types of private health insurance plans. *Group Health Journal* 3:4–11.

Freidson, E. 1960. Client control and medical practice. *American Journal of Sociology* 65:374–82.

———. 1961. *Patients' Views of Medical Practice: A Study of Subscribers to a Prepaid Medical Plan in the Bronx.* New York: Russell Sage Foundation.

———. 1970. *Profession of Medicine: A Study of the Sociology of Applied Knowledge.* New York: Dodd, Mead.

————. 1973. Prepaid group practice and the new "demanding patient." *Milbank Memorial Fund Quarterly / Health and Society* 51:473–88.

————. 1975. *Doctoring Together: A Study of Professional Social Control.* New York: Elsevier.

————. 1985. The reorganization of the medical profession. *Medical Care Review* 42:11–20.

Freidson, E., and J. H. Mann. 1971. Organizational dimensions of large scale group medical practice. *American Journal of Public Health* 61:786–95.

Fretwell, M. D., C. Cutler, and A. M. Epstein. 1987. Outpatient geriatric assessment in a health maintenance organization: Its structure, practice, and clinical implications. *Clinics in Geriatric Medicine* 3:185–91.

Galiher, C. B., and M. A. Costa. 1975. Consumer acceptance of HMOs. *Public Health Reports* 90:106–12.

Gallup Organization, The. 1991. *A National Survey of U.S. Health Plan Consumers.* Final Report. Houston, Tex.: Gallup Organization.

Gellman, R. M. 1986. Divided loyalties: A physician's responsibilities in an information age. *Social Science and Medicine* 23:817–26.

Gerst, A., L. Rogson, and R. Hetherington. 1969. Patterns of satisfaction with health plan coverage: A conceptual approach. *Inquiry* 6:37–51.

Gilman, T. A., and C. K. Bucco. 1987. Alternative delivery systems: An overview. *Topics in Health Care Financing* 13:1–7.

Goldberg, L. G., and W. Greenberg. 1981. The determinants of HMO enrollment and growth. *Health Services Research* 16:421–38.

Goodman, L. J., and J. E. Swartwout. 1984. Comparative aspects of medical practice: Organizational setting and financial arrangements in four delivery systems. *Medical Care* 22:255–67.

Gordon, N. P., and G. A. Kaplan. 1991. Some evidence refuting the HMO "favorable selection" hypothesis: The case of Kaiser Permanente. In Hornbrook, ed., *Risk-based Contributions*, pp. 19–39. *See* Hornbrook 1991.

Goss, M. E. W. 1961. Influence and authority among physicians in an outpatient clinic. *American Sociological Review* 26:39–50.

Gray, B. H., ed. 1986. *For-Profit Enterprise in Health Care.* Washington, D.C.: National Academy Press.

Grazier, K. L., W. C. Richardson, D. P. Martin, and P. Diehr. 1986. Factors affecting choice of health care plans. *Health Services Research* 20:659–82.

Greenberg, I. G., and M. L. Rodburg. 1971. The role of prepaid group practice in relieving the medical care crisis. *Harvard Law Review* 842:887–1001.

Greenberg, J. N., W. Leutz, M. Greenlick, J. Malone, S. Ervin, and D. Kodner. 1988. The social HMO demonstration: Early experience. *Health Affairs* 7:66–79.

Greenlick, M. R. 1971. Medical services to poverty groups. In *The Kaiser Permanente Medical Care Program: A Symposium,* edited by A. B. Somers, pp. 38–51. New York: Commonwealth Fund.

————. 1972. The impact of prepaid group practice on American medical care: A critical evaluation. *American Academy of Political and Social Science Annals* 399:100–113.

————. 1988. Profit and nonprofit organizations in health care: A sociological perspective. In *In Sickness and in Health: The Mission of Voluntary Health Care Institutions,* edited by J. D. Seay and B. C. Vladeck, pp. 155–76. New York: McGraw-Hill.

————. 1989. Health care for adults. In *Handbook of Medical Sociology,* edited by H. E. Freeman and S. Levine, pp. 381–99. Englewood Cliffs, N.J.: Prentice-Hall.

————. 1992. Educating physicians for population-based clinical practice. *JAMA* 267:1645–48.

Greenlick, M. R., D. K. Freeborn, T. J. Colombo, J. A. Prussin, and E. W. Saward. 1972. Comparing the use of medical care services by a medically indigent and a general membership population in a comprehensive prepaid group practice program. *Medical Care* 10:187–200.

Greenlick, M. R., D. K. Freeborn, and C. R. Pope. 1988. *Health Care Research in an HMO: Two Decades of Discovery.* Baltimore: Johns Hopkins University Press.

Greenlick, M. R., A. V. Hurtado, C. R. Pope, E. W. Saward, and S. S. Yoshioka. 1968. Determinants of medical care utilization. *Health Services Research* 3:296–315.

Greenlick, M. R., S. J. Lamb, T. M. Carpenter, Jr., T. S. Fischer, S. D. Marks, and W. J. Cooper. 1983. Kaiser Permanente's Medical Plus Project: A successful prospective payment demonstration. *Health Care Financing Review* 4:85–97.

Griffith, M. J., N. Baloff, and E. L. Spitznagel. 1984. Utilization patterns of health maintenance organization disenrollees. *Medical Care* 22:827–34.

Gruber, L., M. Shadle, M. Porter, and P. Ball. 1990. *The InterStudy Edge.* Vol. 2. Excelsior, Minn.: InterStudy Center for Managed Care Research.

Hadley, J. P., and K. Langwell. 1991. Managed care in the United States: Promises, evidence to date, and future directions. *Health Policy* 19:91–118.

Hale, J. A., and M. M. Hunter. 1988. *From HMO Movement to Managed Care Industry: The Future of HMOs in a Volatile Health Care Market.* Excelsior, Minn.: InterStudy Center for Managed Care Research.

Hall, J. A., and M. C. Dornan. 1988a. Meta-analysis of satisfaction with medical care: Description of research domain and analysis of overall satisfaction levels. *Social Science and Medicine* 27:637–44.

————. 1988b. What patients like about their medical care and how often they are asked: A meta-analysis of the satisfaction literature. *Social Science and Medicine* 27:935–39.

————. 1990. Patient sociodemographic characteristics as predictors of satisfaction with medical care: A meta-analysis. *Social Science and Medicine* 30:811–18.

Hall, J. A., M. Feldstein, M. D. Fretwell, J. W. Rowe, and A. M. Epstein. 1990. Older patients' health status and satisfaction with medical care in an HMO population. *Medical Care* 28:261–70.

Hall, R. H. 1977. *Organizations: Structures and Process.* 2d ed. Englewood Cliffs, N.J.: Prentice-Hall.

Harris, J. M. 1990. Is managed care manageable? *Group Practice Journal* 39:13–16.

Held, D. J., and U. E. Reinhardt. 1980. Prepaid medical practice: A summary of findings from a recent survey of group practices in the United States. *Group Health Journal* 1:4–15.

Hennelly, V. D., and S. B. Boxerman. 1983. Disenrollment from a prepaid group plan: A multivariate analysis. *Medical Care* 21:1154–67.

Hetherington, R. W., C. E. Hopkins, and M. I. Roemer. 1975. *Health Insurance Plans: Promise and Performance.* New York: John Wiley and Sons.

Hibbard, J. H., and E. C. Weeks. 1989. Does the dissemination of comparative data on physician fees affect consumer use of services? *Medical Care* 27:1167–74.

Hornbrook, M. C., ed. 1991. *Risk-based Contributions to Private Health Insurance.* Advances in Health Economics and Health Services Research, vol. 12. Greenwich, Conn.: JAI Press.

Hornbrook, M. C., and S. E. Berki. 1985. Practice mode and payment method: Effects on use, costs, quality, and access. *Medical Care* 23:484–511.

Hornbrook, M. C., and M. J. Goodman. 1991. Managed care: Penalties, autonomy, risk, and integration. In *Primary Care Research: Theory and Methods,* edited by M. L. Grady, pp. 107–26. Rockville, Md.: U.S. Department of Health and Human Services, Agency for Health Care Policy and Research.

Hornbrook, M. C., A. V. Hurtado, and R. E. Johnson. 1985. Health care episodes: Definition, measurement, and use. *Medical Care Review* 42:163–218.

Hosek, S. D., and M. S. Marquis. 1990. *Participation and Satisfaction in Employer Plans with Preferred Provider Organization Options.* Santa Monica, Calif.: RAND Corporation.

Hoy, E. W., R. E. Curtis, and T. Rice. 1991. Change and growth in managed care. *Health Affairs* 10:18–36.

Hudes, J., C. A. Young, L. Sohrab, and C. N. Trinh. 1980. Are HMO enrollees being attracted by a liberal maternity benefit? *Medical Care* 18:635–48.

Hulka, B. S., and J. R. Wheat. 1985. Patterns of utilization: The patient perspective. *Medical Care* 23:438–60.

Hurtado, A. V., and M. R. Greenlick. 1971. A disease classification system for analysis of medical care utilization, with a note on symptom classification. *Health Services Research* 6:235–50.

Iglehart, J. K. 1992a. The American health care system: Managed care. *New England Journal of Medicine* 327:742–47.

———. 1992b. The American health care system: Introduction. *New England Journal of Medicine* 326:962–67.

Jacobs, M. O., and P. D. Mott. 1987. Physician characteristics and training emphasis considered desirable by leaders of HMOs. *Journal of Medical Education* 62:725–31.

Jensen, J. 1992. HMOs outscore both PPOs, traditional indemnity plans in degree of customer satisfaction. *Modern Healthcare* 22:42.

Jonas, S. 1992. *An Introduction to the U.S. Health Care System.* 3d ed. New York: Springer Publishing Co.

Juba, D. A., J. R. Lave, and J. Shaddy. 1980. An analysis of the choice of health benefits plans. *Inquiry* 17:62–71.

Kaiser Foundation Hospitals, Health Services Research Center. 1975a. *Current Membership Study, 1975 Annual Report.* Survey Series HPB Report no. 3. Portland, Ore.: Kaiser Foundation Health Plan of Oregon.

———. 1975b. *Terminations Study, Cumulative Report, October 1974–December 1975.* Survey Series HPA Report no. 5. Portland, Ore.: Kaiser Foundation Health Plan of Oregon.

Kaiser Permanente. 1990. *Statistical Trends.* Oakland: Kaiser Permanente Medical Care Program.

———. 1992. *Facts, 1991–1992,* pp. 1–8. Oakland: Kaiser Permanente Medical Care Program.

Kaiser Permanente Central Office, Department of Medical Economics and Statistics. 1991. "Annual Statistical Review, 1990."

Karasek, R. A. 1979. Job demands, latitude, and mental strain: Implications for job redesign. *Administration Science Quarterly* 24:285–306.

Karasek, R., and T. Theorell. 1990. *Healthy Work: Stress, Productivity, and the Reconstruction of Working Life.* New York: Basic Books.

Katz, D., and R. Kahn. 1978. *The Social Psychology of Organizations.* 2d ed. New York: John Wiley and Sons.

Katz, E., and P. Lazarsfeld. 1955. *Personal Influence.* New York: Free Press.

Katz, L. A. 1992. The crisis in primary care: What it means for HMOs. *HMO Practice* 6:3–5.

Kendrick, M. 1985. PPOs: A challenge to HMOs? *Group Health Journal* 6:22–27.

Kent, C. 1993. Managed care in rural areas: Will the seed take? *Medicine and Health* 47:5–8.

Kindig, D. A., and R. B. Sullivan, eds. 1992. *Understanding Universal Health Programs: Issues and Options.* Ann Arbor: Health Administration Press.

Klinkman, M. S. 1991. The process of choice of health plan and provider: Development of an integrated analytic framework. *Medical Care Review* 48:295–329.

Knickman, J. R., and K. E. Thorpe. 1990. Financing for health care. In Kovner, ed., *Health Care Delivery in the United States,* pp. 240–69. *See* Banta 1990a.

Koehler, W. F., M. D. Fottler, and J. E. Swan. 1992. Physician-patient satisfaction: Equity in the health services encounter. *Medical Care Review* 49:455–84.

Kongstvedt, P. R., ed. 1989. *The Managed Health Care Handbook.* Rockville, Md.: Aspen Publishers.

Kramer, A. M., P. D. Fox, and N. Morgenstern. 1992. Geriatric care approaches in health maintenance organizations. *Journal of the American Geriatric Society* 40:1055–67.

Kraus, N., M. Porter, and P. Ball. 1991. *Managed Care: A Decade in Review, 1980–1990*. Excelsior, Minn.: InterStudy Center for Managed Care Research.

Kravitz, R. L., L. S. Linn, and M. F. Shapiro. 1990. Physician satisfaction under the Ontario Health Insurance Plan. *Medical Care* 28:502–12.

Ku, L., and D. Fisher. 1990. The attitudes of physicians toward health care cost-containment policies. *Health Services Research* 25:25–42.

Kuder, J., and G. Levitz. 1985. Visits to the physician: An evaluation of the usual source effect. *Health Services Research* 20:579–96.

Lairson, D. R., and J. A. Herd. 1987. The role of health practices, health status, and prior health care claims in HMO selection bias. *Inquiry* 24:276–84.

Larsen, D. E., and I. Rootman. 1976. Physician role performance and patient satisfaction. *Social Science and Medicine* 10:29–32.

Lawrence, R. S., and S. Jonas. 1990. Ambulatory care. In Kovner, ed., *Health Care Delivery in the United States*, pp. 106–8. See Banta 1990a.

Lee, R. I., and L. W. Jones. 1933. *The Fundamentals of Good Medical Care.* Chicago: University of Chicago Press.

Lewis, C. E., R. Fein, and D. Mechanic. 1976. *A Right to Health: The Problem of Access to Primary Medical Care*. New York: John Wiley and Sons.

Lewis, K. 1984. Comparison of use by enrolled and recently disenrolled populations in a health maintenance organization. *Health Services Research* 19:1–22.

Lichtenstein, R. L. 1984a. Measuring the job satisfaction of physicians in organized settings. *Medical Care* 22:56–68.

———. 1984b. The job satisfaction and retention of physicians in organized settings: A literature review. *Medical Care Review* 41:139–79.

Lichtenstein, R., J. W. Thomas, J. Adams-Watson, J. Lepkowski, and B. Simone. 1991. Selection bias in TEFRA at-risk HMOs. *Medical Care* 29:318–31.

Like, R., and S. J. Zyzanski. 1987. Patient satisfaction with the clinical encounter: Social psychological determinants. *Social Science and Medicine* 24:351–57.

Linn, L., R. Brook, V. Clark, A. Davies, A. Fink, and J. Kosecoff. 1985. Physician and patient satisfaction as factors related to the organization of internal medicine group practices. *Medical Care* 23:1171–78.

Lochman, J. E. 1983. Factors related to patients' satisfaction with their medical care. *Journal of Community Health* 9:91–109.

Long, S. H., R. F. Settle, and C. W. Wrightson. 1988. Employee premiums, availability of alternative plans, and HMO disenrollment. *Medical Care* 26:927–38.

Louis Harris and Associates. 1980. *American Attitudes toward Health Maintenance Organizations*. Menlo Park, Calif.: Henry J. Kaiser Family Foundation.

———. 1985. *A Report Card on HMOs, 1980–1984*. Summary report. Menlo Park, Calif.: Henry J. Kaiser Family Foundation.

Luft, H. S. 1978. How do health maintenance organizations achieve their "savings"? *New England Journal of Medicine* 298:1336–43.

———. 1980. Assessing the evidence on HMO performance. *Milbank Memorial Fund Quarterly / Health and Society* 58:501–36.

———. 1981. *Health Maintenance Organizations: Dimensions of Performance.* New York: John Wiley and Sons.

———. 1982. Health maintenance organizations and the rationing of medical care. *Milbank Memorial Fund Quarterly / Health and Society* 60:268–306.

———. 1988. HMOs and the quality of care. *Inquiry* 25:147–56.

Luft, H. S., S. S. Hunt, and S. C. Maerki. 1987. The volume-outcome relationship: Practice-makes-perfect or selective-referral patterns? *Health Services Research* 22:157–82.

Luft, H. S., and R. H. Miller. 1988. Patient selection in a competitive health system. *Health Affairs* 7:97–119.

Luft, H. S., and E. M. Morrison. 1991. Alternative delivery systems. In *Health Services Research: Key to Health Policy,* edited by E. Ginsberg, pp. 195–233. Cambridge: Harvard University Press.

McCall, N. 1983. Utilization of Medicare services outside the health maintenance organization by Medicare beneficiaries: A comparative study. *Group Health Journal* 4:24–33.

McDonald, R. B., and C. L. F. Wilke. 1987. Alternative delivery systems and their impact on physicians. *Topics in Health Care Financing* 13:47–59.

McElrath, D. C. 1961. Perspectives and participation of physicians in prepaid group practice. *American Sociological Review* 26:596–607.

McFarland, B. H., D. K. Freeborn, J. P. Mullooly, and C. R. Pope. 1985. Utilization patterns among long-term enrollees in a prepaid group practice health maintenance organization. *Medical Care* 23:1221–33.

———. 1986. Utilization patterns and mortality of HMO enrollees. *Medical Care* 24:200–208.

McGuire, T. G. 1981. Price and membership in a prepaid group medical practice. *Medical Care* 19:172–83.

McLaughlin, C. P., and A. D. Kaluzny. 1990. Total quality management in health: Making it work. *Health Care Management Review* 15:7–14.

Madison, D. L., and T. R. Konrad. 1988. Large medical group-practice organizations and employed physicians: A relationship in transition. *Milbank Quarterly* 66:240–82.

Manning, W. G., A. Leibowitz, G. A. Goldberg, W. H. Rogers, and J. P. Newhouse. 1984. A controlled trial of the effect of a prepaid group practice on use of services. *New England Journal of Medicine* 310:1505–10.

Marquis, M. S. 1983. Consumers' knowledge about their health insurance coverage. *Health Care Financing Review* 5:65–79.

Mawardi, B. H. 1979. Satisfactions, dissatisfactions, and causes of stress in medical practice. *JAMA* 241:1483–86.

Mechanic, D. 1972. General medical practice: Some comparisons between the work of primary care physicians in the United States and England and Wales. *Medical Care* 10:402–20.

———. 1975. The organization of medical practice and practice orientation among physicians in prepaid and nonprepaid primary care settings. *Medical Care* 13:189–204.

———. 1976. *The Growth of Bureaucratic Medicine: An Inquiry into the Dynamics of Patient Behavior and the Organization of Medical Care.* New York: John Wiley and Sons.

———. 1978. *Medical Sociology.* 2d ed. New York: Free Press.

———. 1986. *From Advocacy to Allocation: The Evolving American Health Care System.* New York: Free Press.

———. 1989. Consumer choice among health care options. *Health Affairs* 8:138–48

Mechanic, D., T. Ettel, and D. Davis. 1990. Choosing among health insurance options: A study of new employees. *Inquiry* 27:14–23.

Meir, E. I., and K. Engel. 1986. Interests and specialty choice in medicine. *Social Science and Medicine* 23:527–30.

Melville, A. 1980. Job satisfaction in general practice: Implications for prescribing. *Social Science and Medicine* 14A:495–99.

Merrill, J., C. Jackson, and J. Reuter. 1985. Factors that affect the HMO enrollment decision: A tale of two cities. *Inquiry* 22:388–95.

Merton, R. K. 1968. *Social Structure and Social Theory.* New York: Free Press.

Metzner, C. A., and R. L. Bashshur. 1967. Factors associated with choice of health care plans. *Journal of Health and Social Behavior* 8:291–99.

Metzner, C. A., R. L. Bashshur, and G. W. Shannon. 1972. Differential public acceptance of group medical practice. *Medical Care* 10:279–87.

Mick, S. S., S. Sussman, L. Anderson-Selling, C. DelNero, R. Glazer, E. Hirsch, and D. S. Rowe. 1983. Physician turnover in eight New England prepaid group practices: An analysis. *Medical Care* 21:323–37.

Miller, R. H., and H. S. Luft. 1991. Diversity and transition in health insurance plans. *Health Affairs* 10:37–47.

Moran, D. W., and P. R. Wolfe. 1991. Can managed care control costs? *Health Affairs* 10:120–28.

Morgenstern, H., S. M. Horwitz, and L. F. Berkman. 1986. A prospective study of medical care utilization and morbidity in preschool children belonging to a prepaid group practice: Background and methods. *Yale Journal of Biology and Medicine* 59:599–611.

Morrisey, M. A., and C. S. Ashby. 1982. An empirical analysis of HMO market share. *Inquiry* 19:136–49.

Morrison, E. M., and H. S. Luft. 1990. Health maintenance organization environments in the 1980s and beyond. *Health Care Financing Review* 12:81–90.

Mott, P. E. 1972. *The Characteristics of Effective Organizations.* New York: Harper and Row.

Moustafa, A. T., C. E. Hopkins, and B. Klein. 1971. Determinants of choice and change of health insurance plan. *Medical Care* 9:32–41.

Muller, C. 1986. Review of twenty years of research on medical care utilization. *Health Services Research* 21:129–44.

Mullooly, J. D., and D. K. Freeborn. 1979. The effect of length of membership upon the utilization of ambulatory care services. *Medical Care* 17:922–36.

Murray, J. P. 1987. A comparison of patient satisfaction among prepaid and fee-for-service patients. *Journal of Family Practice* 24:203–7.

———. 1988. A follow-up comparison of patient satisfaction among prepaid and fee-for-service patients. *Journal of Family Practice* 26:576–81.

Murray, T. H. 1986. Divided loyalties for physicians: Social context and moral problems. *Social Science and Medicine* 23:827–32.

Nash, D. B. 1988. Physician satisfaction and HMOs. *HMO Practice* 2:1.

National Center for Health Statistics (NCHS). 1992. *Health, United States, 1991.* DHHS Publication PHS 91-1232. Washington, D.C.: U.S. Government Printing Office.

Navarro, V. 1988. Professional dominance or proletarianization? Neither. *Milbank Quarterly* 66 (suppl. 2): 57–75.

Nelson, L. M., K. M. Langwell, and R. S. Brown. 1987–88. Comparison of "rollovers" and "switchers" among enrollees of Medicare HMOs. *GHAA Journal* 8:63–78.

Parsons, E. M., and M. I. Roemer. 1976. Ideological goals of different health insurance plans. *Journal of Community Health* 1:241–48.

Parsons, T. 1951. *The Social System.* New York: Free Press.

Pasternak, D. P., W. C. Tuttle, and H. L. Smith. 1986. Physician satisfaction in group practice: A comparison of primary care physicians with specialists. *GHAA Journal* 7:50–59.

Patrick, D. L., and P. Erickson. 1993. *Health Status and Health Policy: Quality of Life in Health Care Evaluation and Resource Allocation.* New York: Oxford University Press.

Pauly, M. V., A. L. Hillman, and J. Kerstein. 1990. Managing physician incentives in managed care: The role of for-profit ownership. *Medical Care* 28:1013–24.

Phillips, K. 1987. Self-selection factors in choosing a health plan. *Business and Health* 4:29–30.

Pineault, R. 1976. The effect of prepaid group practice on physicians' utilization behavior. *Medical Care* 14:121–36.

———. 1985. The physician episode of care: A framework for analyzing physician behavior regarding use of clinical and technical resources. *Clinical and Investigative Medicine* 8:48–55.

Piontkowski, D., and L. Butler. 1980. Selection of health insurance by an employee group in Northern California. *American Journal of Public Health* 70:274–76.

Pope, C. R. 1978. Consumer satisfaction in a health maintenance organization. *Journal of Health and Social Behavior* 19:291–303.

Pope, C. R., D. K. Freeborn, and S. Marks. 1984. Perceived access to care and patient satisfaction in a prepaid group practice HMO. *Group Health Journal* 584:22–28.

Porter, M. J., and P. A. Ball. 1992. *The InterStudy Competitive Edge.* Vol. 2, no. 1. Excelsior, Minn.: InterStudy Center for Managed Care Research.

Povar, G., and J. Moreno. 1988. Hippocrates and the health maintenance organization: A discussion of ethical issues. *Annals of Internal Medicine* 109:419–24.

Priest, D. 1993. Health care organizations back national database to rate their plans. *Washington Post,* January 15.

Prybil, L. D. 1971. Physician terminations in large multispecialty groups. *Medical Group Management* 18:5–6.

———. 1974. Characteristics, career patterns, and opinions of physicians who practice in large multi-specialty groups. *Medical Group Management* 21:22–26.

Reames, H. R., and D. C. Dunstone. 1989. Professional satisfaction of physicians. *Archives of Internal Medicine* 149:1951–56.

Relman, A. S. 1992a. What market values are doing to medicine. *Atlantic Monthly* 269:99–106.

———. 1992b. Reforming our health care system: A physician's perspective. *Key Reporter* 58:1–5.

Relman, A. S., and U. Reinhardt. 1986. An exchange on for-profit health care. In *For-Profit Enterprise in Health Care,* edited by B. H. Gray, pp. 209–23. Washington, D.C.: Institute of Medicine, National Academy Press.

Rice, T. 1992. Containing health care costs in the United States. *Medical Care Review* 49:19–65.

Richardson, W. C., P. K. Diehr, J. P. LoGerfo, K. M. McCaffree, and S. M. Shortell. 1980. *Comparisons of Prepaid Health Care Plans in a Competitive Market: The Seattle Prepaid Health Care Project.* National Center for Health Services Research (NCHSR) Research Summary Series. Washington, D.C.: U.S. Department of Health and Human Services.

Robertson, E. M. 1993. What does it take to make a member highly satisfied? *Kaiser Permanente Spectrum,* Fall, pp. 22, 23.

Robert Wood Johnson Foundation. 1978. "Special Report," no. 1. Princeton, N.J.: Office of Information Services.

Robinson, J. C., L. B. Gardner, and H. S. Luft. 1993. Health plan switching in anticipation of increased medical care utilization. *Medical Care* 31:43–51.

Roghmann, K. J., J. W. Gavett, A. A. Sorensen, S. Wells, and R. Wersinger. 1975. Who chooses prepaid medical care: Survey results from two marketings of three new prepayment plans. *Public Health Reports* 90:516–27.

Rosenberg, D., P. G. Bonner, D. J. Scotti, and A. R. Wiman. 1989. HMO reenrollment determinants: A multivariate revisit. *Journal of Health and Human Resources Administration* 11:389–95.

Rosko, M. D., and R. W. Broyles. 1988. *The Economics of Health Care: A Reference Handbook.* New York: Greenwood Press.

Ross, A. 1969. A report on physician terminations in group practice. *Medical Group Management* 16:15–21.

Ross, C. E., J. Mirowsky, and R. S. Duff. 1982. Physician status characteristics and client satisfaction in two types of medical practice. *Journal of Health and Social Behavior* 23:317–29.

Rossiter, L. F., K. Langwell, T. T. H. Wan, and M. Rivnyak. 1989. Patient satisfaction among elderly enrollees and disenrollees in Medicare health maintenance organizations: Results from the national Medicare competition evaluation. *JAMA* 262:57–63.

Rubin, H. R., B. Gandek, W. H. Rogers, M. Kosinski, C. A. McHorney, and J. E. Ware, Jr. 1993. Patients' ratings of outpatient visits in different practice settings. *JAMA* 270:835–40.

Saward, E. W. 1970. The relevance of the Kaiser-Permanente experience to the health services of the eastern United States. *Bulletin of the New York Academy of Medicine* 46:707–17.

Saward, E. W., J. D. Blank, and M. R. Greenlick. 1968. Documentation of twenty years of operation and growth of a prepaid group practice plan. *Medical Care* 6:231–44.

Saward, E. W., J. D. Blank, and H. Lamb. 1973. *Some Information Descriptive of a Successfully Operating HMO*, p. 2. Department of Health, Education, and Welfare, Publication (HSM) 73-13011. Washington, D.C.: U.S. Government Printing Office.

Saward, E. W., and M. R. Greenlick. 1972. Health policy and the HMO. *Milbank Memorial Fund Quarterly* 50:147–76.

Scheckler, W. E., and R. Schulz. 1987. Rapid change to HMO systems: Profile of the Dane County, Wisconsin, experience. *Journal of Family Practice* 24:417–24.

Schlesinger, M. 1986. On the limits of expanding health care reform: Chronic care in prepaid settings. *Milbank Quarterly* 64:189–215.

Schmoldt, R. A. 1991. Physician burnout in a prepaid group practice health maintenance organization. Ph.D. diss., University of Minnesota.

Schulz, R., W. Scheckler, C. Girard, and K. Barker. 1990. Physician adaptation to health maintenance organizations and implications for management. *Health Services Research* 25:43–64.

Schulz, R., and C. Schulz. 1988. Management practices, physician autonomy, and satisfaction: Evidence from mental health institutions in the Federal Republic of Germany. *Medical Care* 26:750–63.

Scitovsky, A. A., L. Benham, and N. McCall. 1981. Out-of-plan use under two prepaid plans. *Medical Care* 19:1165–93.

Scitovsky, A. A., N. McCall, and L. Benham. 1978. Factors affecting the choice between two prepaid plans. *Medical Care* 16:660–81.

Scott, W. R. 1966. Professionals in bureaucracies—areas of conflict. In *Professionalization*, edited by H. M. Vollmer and D. L. Mills, pp. 265–75. Englewood Cliffs, N.J.: Prentice-Hall.

———. 1990. Innovation in medical care organizations: A synthetic review. *Medical Care Review* 47:165–92.

Scott, W. R., and S. M. Shortell. 1988. Organizational performance: Managing for efficiency and effectiveness. In *Health Care Management*, 2d ed., edited by

S. M. Shortell and A. Kaluzny, pp. 418–57. New York: John Wiley and Sons.

Shapiro, S. 1984. Review of twenty years of research on HMOs. Proceedings of the Twentieth Anniversary Research Symposium, Portland, Ore.

Shapiro, S., H. Jacobziner, P. M. Densen, and L. Weiner. 1960. Further observations on prematurity and perinatal mortality in a general population and in a population of a prepaid group practice medical care plan. *American Journal of Public Health* 50:1304–17.

Shapiro, S. E., L. Weiner, and P. M. Densen. 1958. Comparison of prematurity and perinatal mortality in a general practice population and in the population of a prepaid group practice medical care plan. *American Journal of Public Health* 48:170–87.

Shimshak, D. G., M. C. DeFuria, J. J. DiGiorgio, and J. Getson. 1987. An analysis of HMO disenrollment data. *GHAA Journal* 8:13–22.

———. 1988. Controlling disenrollment in health maintenance organizations. *Health Care Management Review* 13:47–55.

Shortell, S. M. 1991. *Effective Hospital-Physician Relationships.* Ann Arbor: Health Administration Press.

Shortell, S. M., and A. D. Kaluzny. 1988. *Health Care Management: A Text in Organizational Theory and Behavior.* 2d ed. New York: John Wiley and Sons.

Shuttiga, J., M. Falik, and B. Steinwald. 1984. *Health Plan Selection in the Federal Employee Health Benefits Program.* Washington, D.C.: U.S. Department of Health and Human Services.

Sloss, E. M., E. B. Keeler, R. H. Brook, B. H. Operskalski, G. A. Goldberg, and J. P. Newhouse. 1987. Effect of a health maintenance organization on physiologic health: Results from a randomized trial. *Annals of Internal Medicine* 106:130–38.

Smillie, J. G. 1991. *Can Physicians Manage the Quality and Costs of Health Care? The Story of the Permanente Medical Group.* New York: McGraw-Hill.

Smith, D. B., and A. D. Kaluzny. 1986. *The White Labyrinth: A Guide to the Health Care System.* 2d ed. Ann Arbor: Health Administration Press.

Somers, A. R. 1971. *The Kaiser Permanente Medical Care Program.* New York: Commonwealth Fund.

Somers, H. M., and A. R. Somers. 1961. *Doctors, Patients, and Health Insurance: The Organization and Financing of Medical Care.* Washington, D.C.: Brookings Institution.

Sorensen, A. A., and R. P. Wersinger. 1980. Aspects of member satisfaction under two types of health delivery systems. *Group Health Journal* 1:33–41.

———. 1981. Factors influencing disenrollment from an HMO. *Medical Care* 19:766–73.

Staines, V. S. 1993. Potential impact of managed care on national health care spending. *Health Affairs* 12 (suppl.): 248–57.

Starr, P. 1982. *The Social Transformation of American Medicine.* New York: Basic Books.

Stevens, V. J., and M. R. Greenlick. 1989. The HMO as a health promotion laboratory. *HMO Practice* 3:89–94.

Strumpf, G. B., F. H. Seubold, and M. B. Arrill. 1978. Health maintenance organizations, 1971–1977: Issues and answers. *Journal of Community Health* 4:33–54.

Strumwasser, I., N. V. Paranjpe, D. L. Ronis, J. McGinnis, D. W. Kee, and H. L. Hall. 1989. The triple option choice: Self-selection bias in traditional coverage, HMOs, and PPOs. *Inquiry* 26:432–41.

Taylor, H., and M. Kagay. 1986. The HMO report card: A closer look. *Health Affairs* 5:81–89.

Terris, M. 1990. Failing health: A wasteful system that doesn't work. *Progressive* 54:14–16.

Tessler, R., and D. Mechanic. 1975a. Consumer satisfaction with prepaid group practice: A comparative study. *Journal of Health and Social Behavior* 16:95–113.

————. 1975b. Factors affecting the choice between prepaid group practice and alternative insurance programs. *Milbank Memorial Fund Quarterly / Health and Society* 53:149–72.

Thorpe, K. E. 1990. Health care cost containment: Reflections and future directions. In Kovner, ed., *Health Care Delivery in the United States*, pp. 270–96. *See* Banta 1990a.

U.S. Department of Health and Human Services (USDHHS). 1988. *Health, United States, 1987*. DHHS Publication no. PHS 88-1232. Washington, D.C.: U.S. Government Printing Office.

U.S. Department of Health, Education, and Welfare (USDHEW). 1962. *International Classification of Diseases, Adapted*. DHEW, Public Health Service publication 719. Washington, D.C.: U.S. Government Printing Office.

U.S. General Accounting Office (USGAO). 1991. *Health Insurance Coverage: A Profile of the Uninsured in Selected States*. Washington, D.C.: USGAO.

Vogt, T. M. 1993. Paradigms and prevention. *American Journal of Public Health* 83:795–96.

Vohs, J. A., R. V. Anderson, and R. Straus. 1972. Critical issues in HMO strategy. *New England Journal of Medicine* 286:1082–86.

Wallack, S. S. 1991. Managed care: Practice, pitfalls, and potential. *Health Care Financing Review*, annual suppl., pp. 27–34.

Wan, T. T. H. 1989. The effect of managed care on health services use by dually eligible elders. *Medical Care* 27:983–1001.

Ware, J. E., Jr., R. H. Brook, W. H. Rogers, E. B. Keeler, A. R. Davies, C. D. Sherbourne, G. A. Goldberg, P. Camp, and J. P. Newhouse. 1986. Comparison of health outcomes at a health maintenance organization with those of fee-for-service care. *Lancet* 1:1017–22.

Ware, J. E., Jr., A. R. Davies, and H. R. Rubin. 1988. Patients' assessments of their care. In *The Quality of Medical Care: Information for Consumers*, pp. 231–47. OTA-H-386. Washington, D.C.: U.S. Congress, Office of Technology Assessment.

Weinerman, E. R. 1964. Patients' perceptions of group medical care. *American Journal of Public Health* 54:880–89.

————. 1967. Patients' perceptions of group medical care: A review and analysis of studies of choice and utilization of prepaid group practice plans. In *Medical Care in Transition*, pp. 158–67. DHEW Public Health Service. Washington, D.C.: U.S. Government Printing Office.

———. 1969. Problems and perspectives in group practice. *Group Practice* 18:27–32.

Weiss, B. D., and J. H. Senf. 1990. Patient satisfaction survey instrument for use in health maintenance organizations. *Medical Care* 28:434–45.

Welch, W. P. 1985. Regression toward the mean in medical care costs: Implications for biased selection in health maintenance organizations. *Medical Care* 23:1234–41.

———. 1987. The new structure of individual practice associations. *Journal of Health Politics, Policy, and Law* 12:723–39.

Welch, W. P., and R. G. Frank. 1986. The predictors of HMO enrollee populations: Results from a national sample. *Inquiry* 23:16–22.

Welch, W. P., A. L. Hillman, and M. V. Pauly. 1990. Toward new typologies for HMOs. *Milbank Quarterly* 68:221–43.

Wennberg, J. E. 1990. On the status of the prostate disease assessment team. *Health Services Research* 25:709–16.

Wersinger, R. P., and A. A. Sorensen. 1982. Demographic characteristics and prior utilization experience of HMO disenrollees compared with total membership. *Medical Care* 20:1188–96.

Wilensky, G. R., and L. F. Rossiter. 1986. Patient self-selection in HMOs. *Health Affairs* 5:66–80.

Williams, G. 1971. *Kaiser Permanente Health Plan: Why It Works*. Oakland, Calif.: Henry J. Kaiser Foundation.

Williams, S. J., and P. R. Torrens, eds. 1993. *Introduction to Health Services*. 4th ed. Albany, N.Y.: Delmar Publishers.

Winkenwerder, W., and D. B. Nash. 1988. Corporately managed health care and the new role of physicians. *Cancer Investigation* 6:209–17.

Wintringham, K. 1982. Impact of step-rating and price sensitivity on disenrollment and risk selection: The experience of a group practice HMO. *Group Health Journal* 3:15–20.

Wolinsky, F. D. 1976. Health service utilization and attitudes toward health maintenance organizations: A theoretical and methodological discussion. *Journal of Health and Social Behavior* 17:221–36.

———. 1980. The performance of health maintenance organizations: An analytical review. *Milbank Memorial Fund Quarterly / Health and Society* 58:537–87.

———. 1982. Why physicians choose different types of practice settings. *Health Services Research* 17:399–419.

———. 1985. *The Organization of Medical Practice and the Practice of Medicine*. Ann Arbor: Health Administration Press.

Wolinsky, F. D., and W. D. Marder. 1982. Spending time with patients: The impact of organizational structure on medical practice. *Medical Care* 20:1051–59.

————. 1983. The organization of medical practice and primary care physician income. *American Journal of Public Health* 73:379–83.

Wrightson, W., J. Genuardi, and S. Stephens. 1987. Demographic and utilization characteristics of HMO disenrollees. *GHAA Journal* 8:23–42.

Zapka, J. G., E. J. Stanek, and J. Raitt. 1986. HMO disenrollment—who leaves and why?—operational considerations. In *New Health Care Systems: HMOs and Beyond*. Proceedings of the Thirty-sixth Annual Group Health Institute. Washington, D.C.: Group Health Association of America.

Index

Access to care
  appointment lag and waiting time in
    KPNW, 57–59
  and continuity in managed care, 51–
    69
  factors influencing, 54–55
  measurement of, 129
  and members' use of service in
    KPNW, 60
  predictors of, among KPNW
    subscribers, 62–66, 145
  satisfaction of KPNW members with,
    77
  and socioeconomic status, 52, 57, 67–
    68
Adverse selection
  and HMOs, 38–39
  and risk-adjustment, 122
Ambulatory care
  and innovations in HMOs, 127–28
  use of services in, 60–64
American Medical Association
  and acceptance of managed care, 3
  and definition of managed care, 2

Blue Cross and Blue Shield
  origins of, 29
  role of, 14
Bureaucratization
  advantages and disadvantages of, in
    organized medicine, 19
  as source of conflict with professional
    values, 94–96

Choosing managed care
  access factors in, 46–47
  cost and coverage factors in, 43–46
  reasons for, 28–50
Committee on the Costs of Medical
    Care (CCMC), recommendations of,
    13–14
Consumers
  attitudes, values, and behaviors of,
    42–43
  satisfaction of, with medical care, 70–
    92
Continuity of care. See Access to care
Corporate medicine, fears about, 17–19
Cost of care, satisfaction of KPNW
    members with, 75–77

Data sources
  descriptions of, 139–44
  overview of, 9–10
Disenrollees, characteristics of, in
    KPNW, 88–90
Disenrollment
  from HMOs, 90–91
  reasons for, in KPNW, 87–91
Ellwood, Paul, and coining of term
    "HMO," 15
Enthoven, Alain, and "managed
    competition," 3

Favorable selection. See Adverse
  selection

Fee-for-service
  compared to HMOs, 23–25
  as different from managed care, 72
  physician satisfaction with, 117

Gatekeepers
  HMO physicians' attitudes toward
    function of, 113
  role conflicts of, 111
Guidelines
  physicians' views of, 132
  role of, in managed care, 132–33

Health care system, U.S.
  compared to that of other countries, 6
  reform of, 1–2, 120
Health insurance
  choice of, 28–50
  consumer knowledge about, 49–50
  as a fringe benefit, 29
  consumers' need for objective
    information about, 127
  KPNW members' opinions about role
    of government in, 41–42
  KPNW members' self-reported
    knowledge about, 41
  origins of, 14
  role of employers in, 30–31
  types of, 29
Health Maintenance Organization Act
    passage of, 15
  primary objective of, 30
Health maintenance organizations
    (HMOs)
  ability of, to serve diverse populations,
    121–25
  access to preventive care in, 67–68
  advantages and disadvantages of, for
    physicians, 93–94
  advantages of, for members, 3, 15
  ambulatory care in, 127–29
  appointment lags and waiting times
    for members in, 58–59
  attitudes of U.S. physicians toward,
    117
  compared to fee-for-service, 23–25
  continuity and coordination of care in,
    53–54
  disease prevention, health promotion
    in, 124–25, 133

enhancing physician performance and
    satisfaction in, 129
factors influencing access to care in,
    51–52
and "favorable selection," 38–39
growth of, 15, 20–21
improving consumer satisfaction in,
    126
management of chronic disease in,
    124
meeting consumers' needs in, 125
models of, 21–23
origin of name, 15
outside use and disenrollment of
    enrollees in, 89–91
patient satisfaction with, 126
physician autonomy in, 105
physician satisfaction with, 97
physicians' reasons for joining, 101–3
popular images of, 71–72
promise and characteristics of, 20
and quality of care, 24
satisfaction of members with,
    compared to traditional plans, 72
Health plan choice
  conceptualization of process, 31–33
  constraints on, 50
  significant predictors of, in KPNW,
    48–49, 145
Health plans. See Health insurance

Independent practice associations (IPAs),
    as HMO model, 22–24

Kaiser Permanente, Northwest Region
    (KPNW)
  appointment lag and waiting time in,
    57–59
  benefits and services in, 56–57
  characteristics of members in, 49
  choice and access to physician in, 56–
    57, 64–65
  disenrollment from, 87–91
  health status of members in, compared
    to other plans, 38–40
  history and organizational structure
    of, 8–9
  members' reasons for choosing, 43,
    47–48

members' satisfaction with, 70–92, 125–26
members' use of services in, 60–64
perceived effect of membership in, on health status, 39
physicians' satisfaction with, 103–6, 108–15, 125–26
quality of care, as factor in choosing, 47–48
sociodemographic characteristics of members in, compared to other plans, 35–38

Managed care
ability to serve diverse populations, 122–23
access and continuity in, 51–69
choosing, 28–50
consumers in, 125–27
definitions of, 2–4
disease prevention, health promotion in, 133
future of, 120–37
in health care reform, 120–21
history of, 12–17
physician autonomy in, 105
and physician satisfaction with, 93–119
policy issues in, 134–36
recruitment of physicians in, 130–31

Physician, regular
access to, in KPNW, 64–65
in HMO versus fee-for-service, 65–66
Physicians (in KPNW)
characteristics of, 99–100
and reasons for joining, 100
satisfaction of, by specialty, 107–12
satisfaction of, with KPNW, 98–119, 146
and views of KP, compared with other plans, 106–8
and views of patients, 110–11
and views regarding autonomy, 104
Physician satisfaction
and autonomy, 94
factors influencing, 98
in managed care versus fee-for-service, 96–97

with managed care, 93–119
and performance, 118–19
and physician-patient interactions, 97
theoretical model for, 99–100
Preferred Provider Organizations (PPOs)
advantages of, 3
definition and description of, 25–27
promise of, 19–20
Primary care physicians
and gatekeeping role, in HMO versus fee-for-service, 53–54
and problems with roles and practice conditions, in managed care settings, 118
and role conflict in KPNW, 111–12
satisfaction of with KPNW, 108–15

Quality of care and service
as factors in choosing health plan, 47–48
satisfaction of KPNW members with, 79–80

Reinhardt, Uwe, on corporate medicine, 18
Relman, Arnold, on prepaid group practice, 24

Satisfaction, of KPNW members
with access to care, 77–81, 83–87
conceptual framework for examining, 73–74
with cost of care, 75–77
and disenrollment from KPNW, 87–91
with most recent visit, 81–82
predictors of, 146
with quality of care and service, 79–81, 83–87
summary of findings about, 91–92
Shadid, Michael, and history of managed care, 13
Socioeconomic status, and access to care in KPNW, 52, 57, 67–68
Staff-model HMOs, and physician autonomy, 98
Starr, Paul, on future of American medicine, 18

Library of Congress Cataloging-in-Publication Data

Freeborn, Donald K.
  Promise and performance in managed care : the prepaid group practice model /
Donald K. Freeborn and Clyde R. Pope.
    p.   cm.
  Includes bibliographical references and index.
  ISBN 0-8018-4819-9
  1. Health maintenance organizations—United States. 2. Managed
care plans (Medical care)—United States. 3. Health maintenance
organizations—United States—Employees—Attitudes. 4. Patient
satisfaction—United States. I. Pope, Clyde R. II. Title.
RA413.5.U5F74 1994
362.1'0425—dc20   94-6176